101 Vegetarian Weight-Loss RECIPES

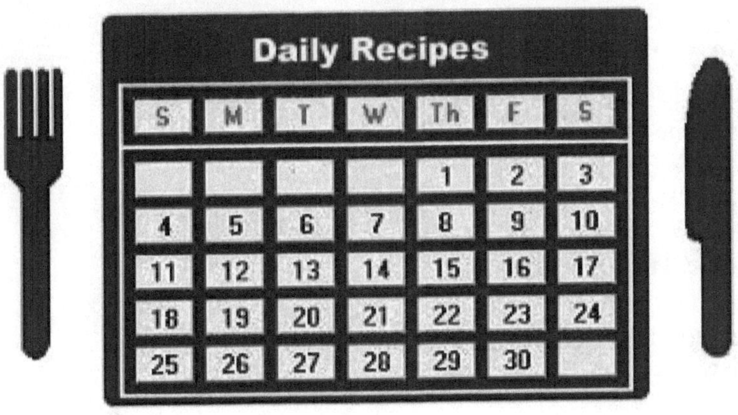

Compiled by NoPaperPress Staff
Edited by Gail Johnson

Recipes by: Gail Johnson, Susan Chen, Charlotte Wise, S. Vijay Gupta and Elena Novak

NoPaperPress™

CONTENTS

Introduction

Our objective at NoPaperPress is to publish fitness, weight control and nutrition eBooks for sensible adults. ***101 Vegetarian Weight Loss Recipes*** is a continuation of that mission. This eBook is a compilation of the best low-calorie recipes from four of our published vegetarian diet eBooks. Most of the101 low-calorie vegetarian recipes are intended for the evening meal. And most, but not all, the recipes serve four. All the recipes specify the calorie value per serving. All the recipes are between 250 and 550 Calories - and all are delicious. The recipes are grouped as follows:
– Low-Calorie Vegetarian-based Recipes (8)
– Low-Calorie Tofu Recipes (27)
– Low-Calorie Soup Recipes (45)
– Low-Calorie Vegetarian Seafood Recipes (48)
– Low-Calorie Vegetarian Pasta & Pizza Recipes (79)
– Low-Calorie Salad Recipes (102)

As mentioned, most often the recipes in this eBook only cover the evening meal. To lose weight you should monitor what you eat the remainder of the day. In this regard, we recommend the 90-Day Vegetarian Diet. The eBook is published by NoPaperPress and has 90 Daily Meal Plans with low-calorie vegetarian recipes.

Note that the recipes in this eBook are a popular vegetarian variant called **Pesceterian**, because the diet includes seafood, eggs and dairy products. Of course Pesceterians do not eat meat or poultry. The inclusion of seafood and eggs assures that your intake of protein will be more than adequate. People often adopt a Pescetarian diet for health reasons, or as a stepping stone to a fully vegetarian diet.

Recipe 1

<u>Wild Rice & Quinoa Mix with Veggies</u>

 ¼ cup wild rice, dry
 ½ cup quinoa, dry
 1 bunch Kale (about 1 lb)
 2 medium sweet potatoes, cut in
 8 medium button mushrooms
 2 tablespoons olive oil, divided

1. Cook wild rice and quinoa according to package directions.
2. Clean and quarter mushrooms. Over medium heat sauté mushrooms in olive oil until they turn reddish brown with golden spots, about 10 minutes.
3. Cut sweet potatoes into bite-size pieces. Place in baking pan and coat potatoes lightly with olive oil. Roast in oven set at 375°F for about 25 minutes, or until done.
4. Wash kale and remove kale stems. Chop and then steam until tender.
5. Plate and serve hot.

<u>Serves 4</u>. About 270 Calories per serving

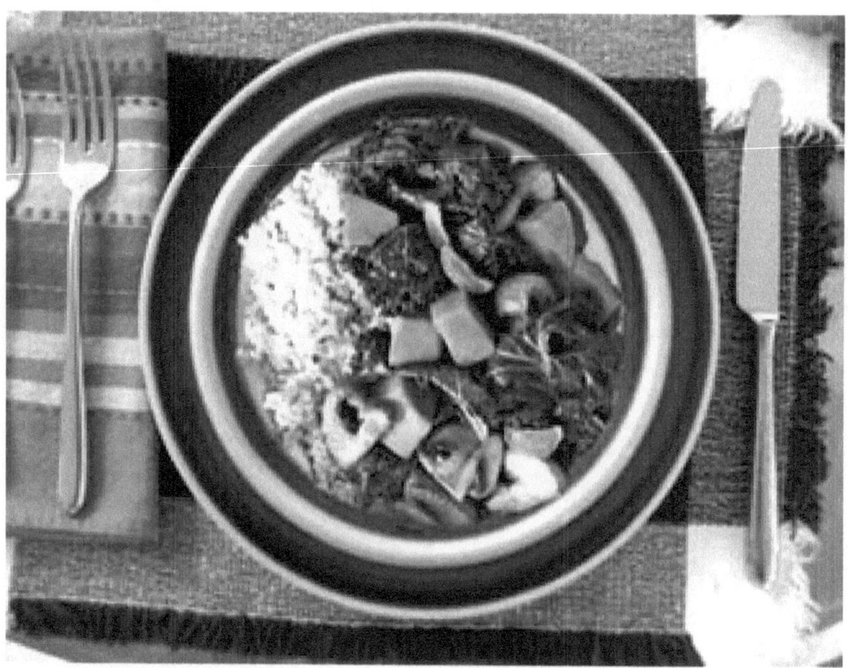

Note: Add a small whole-grain roll which brings the total for the meal to 350 Calories.

Recipe 2

<u>Vegetable Chili</u>

- 1 tablespoon olive oil
- 2 medium carrots, in ½-inch pieces
- 2 medium parsnips, in ½-inch pieces
- 1 medium onion, chopped
- 2 cans (15-ounces each) red kidney beans, drained
- 4 teaspoons chili powder
- 1 can (28-ounce) whole tomatoes in juice
- ¼ cup fresh cilantro leaves, chopped

In saucepot, heat olive oil on medium-high. Add carrots, parsnips, chopped onion, and cook 6 to 8 minutes or until all vegetables are tender and beginning to brown, stirring occasionally.

Meanwhile, on large plate, mash 1 cup drained beans. Stir chili powder into vegetables in saucepot; cook 1 minute, stirring. Add canned tomatoes with their juice, whole and mashed beans, and 2 cups water. Heat to boiling on high, breaking up tomatoes with spoon. Reduce heat to medium and cook, uncovered for 10 minutes, stirring occasionally. Finally, stir in cilantro and serve.

<u>Serves 4</u>.   360 Calories per serving

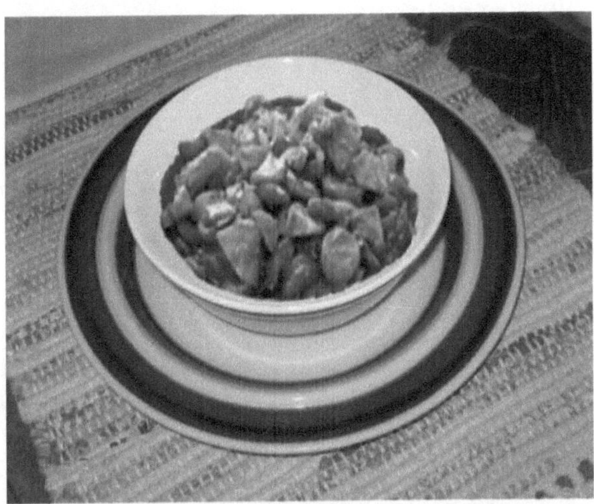

Note: Serve the chili with ½ cup of cooked brown rice which adds about 130 Calories. Then the total for this healthy meal would be 490 Calories.

Recipe 3

<u>Hearty Lentil Stew</u>

  ½ cup chopped onion
  2 garlic cloves, minced
  1 tablespoon vegetable oil
  1 cup lentils, rinsed
  4 tsp vegetable or chicken bouillon granules
  3 tsp Worcestershire sauce
  1 bay leaf
  1 cup chopped carrots
14.5-ounce can diced tomatoes with liquid
10-oz package frozen chopped spinach, thawed
  1 Tbsp red wine vinegar

In a large saucepan, sauté onion and garlic in oil until tender. Add 5 cups of water, lentils, bouillon, Worcestershire sauce, ½ teaspoon salt, ¼ teaspoon black pepper and the bay leaf. Bring to a boil. Reduce heat; cover and simmer for 20 minutes.

Add the carrots, tomatoes and spinach; return to a boil. Reduce heat; cover and simmer additional 15 to 20 minutes, or until lentils are tender. Stir in vinegar and serve.

<u>**Serves 4**</u>. 260 Calories per serving

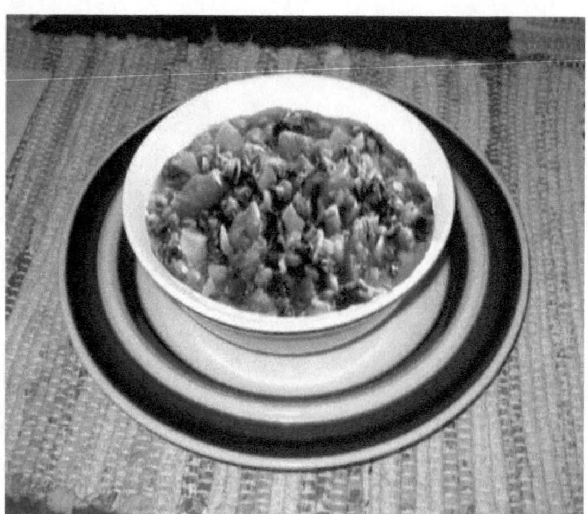

Note: Serve the stew with a large tossed salad (with 1½ tablespoons of low-calorie dressing). This adds about 70 Calories. Then the total for this meal is 330 Calories.

Recipe 4

<u>Black-Eyed Peas over Rice</u>

    2 cups fat-free vegetable broth
    2 cups water
    ½ teaspoon kosher salt
    ½ teaspoon freshly ground black pepper
    1-pound bag frozen black-eyed peas, thawed
    12-ounce bunch fresh turnip greens, trimmed and coarsely chopped
    2 tablespoons pepper vinegar

Cook bacon in a Dutch oven over medium heat until crisp. Remove bacon from pan using a slotted spoon, reserving drippings in pan. Crumble bacon.

Add onion to drippings in pan; sauté 4 minutes, stirring occasionally. Stir in broth and the next 5 ingredients (through greens); bring to a boil. Reduce heat, and simmer for about an hour or until peas are tender, stirring occasionally and skimming as necessary. Stir in vinegar. Ladle about 1⅓ cups pea mixture into each of 4 bowls and top evenly with crumbled bacon.

<u>Serves 4</u>. 380 Calories per serving (includes ½ cup cooked brown rice)

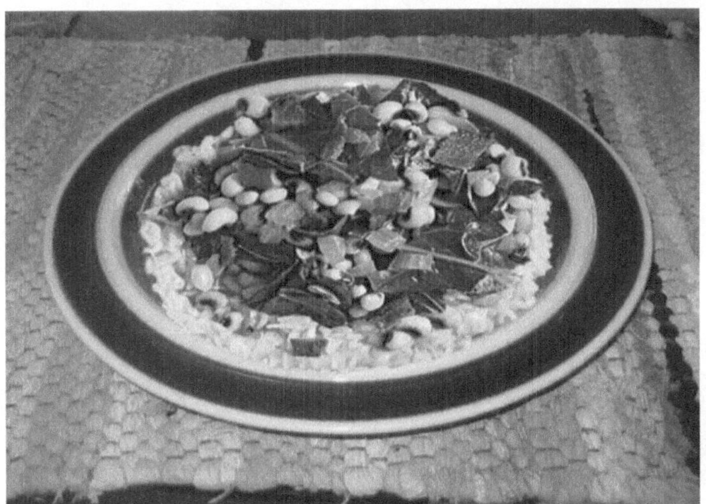

Two servings of black-eyed peas over brown rice on platter.

* Photo shows bacon chips which obviously don't belong in this meal!

Recipe 5

<u>Polenta-Stuffed Peppers</u>

   4 plum tomatoes, halved
   1 red onion, cut into wedges
   1 tablespoon olive oil
   4 poblano peppers, halved lengthwise
   ¼ teaspoon ground cinnamon
   ½ cup polenta
   1 10-ounce package frozen corn
   ¼ cup soft goat cheese (2 ounces)
   4 scallions, sliced

1. Heat broiler. On a rimmed baking sheet, toss the tomatoes, onion, and oil. Turn tomatoes cut-side down. Add the peppers, cut-side down. Broil until tender and charred, stirring the onions and turning tomatoes and peppers halfway through, 5 to 8 minutes.
2. Heat oven to 400° F. In a food processor, puree tomatoes, onion, cinnamon, ½ teaspoon salt, and ¼ teaspoon pepper until smooth. Spread half the sauce in a 9-by-13-inch baking dish. Arrange the peppers in the dish, cut-side up.
3. In a medium saucepan, bring 2¼ cups water to a boil. Add ½ teaspoon salt. Gradually whisk in polenta. Cook, whisking constantly, until thickened, 3 to 4 minutes. Stir in corn, cheese, and all but 2 tablespoons of the scallions.
4. Divide the polenta among peppers. Top with remaining sauce and bake until heated through, 5 to 10 minutes. Sprinkle with the remaining scallions before serving.
<u>Serves 4.</u>   290 Calories per serving

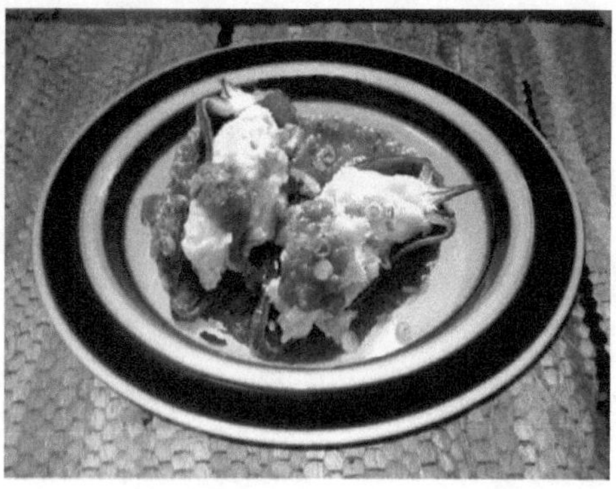

Note: Serve with a large tossed salad (with 1½ tablespoons of low-calorie dressing) and a small whole-grain roll. This adds about 150 Calories. Then the total for this meal is 440 Calories

Recipe 6

<u>Mexican Rice and Beans</u>

 1 cup brown rice
 ½ small onion, diced
 2 garlic cloves, minced
 2 tablespoons olive oil
 1 14½-ounce can diced tomatoes
 1 15-ounce can black beans, rinsed and drained
 1 medium fresh jalapeño, cored and finely chopped
 ½ cup finely chopped fresh oregano and cilantro leaves
 ½ teaspoon cumin, salt & pepper

1. In 1-quart saucepan, combine rice with 2 cups cold water. Bring to boil over medium-high heat, cover, reduce heat to low, and cook for 20 minutes. Remove from heat and let pan stand, covered, for another 5 minutes.

2. While rice steams, set a fine sieve over bowl and drain can of tomatoes. Pour tomato juices into a 1-cup liquid measure. Add enough water to tomato juices to equal 1 cup.

3. Heat a 10- to 12-inch skillet over medium-high heat. Pour in oil and stir-fry garlic and jalapeño until garlic browns and jalapeño smells pungent, about 1 minute. Add black beans, salt, and cumin; stir three times to incorporate mixture. Cook about 30 seconds.

4. Stir in tomato juice and water mixture and bring to a boil. Adjust heat to maintain a gentle boil and cook, stirring occasionally, until beans absorb much of liquid, about 6 minutes. Add tomatoes, oregano, cilantro, and cooked rice and cook, stirring occasionally, until rice is warm, about 2 minutes. Serve immediately.

<u>**Serves 6.**</u> About 270 Calories per serving

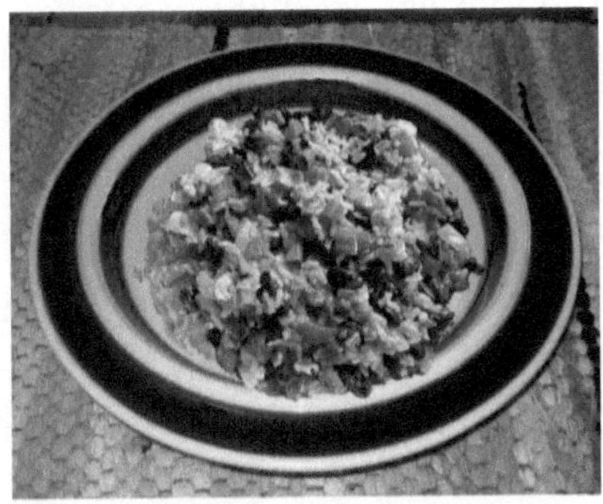

Note: Serve the rice and beans with a large tossed salad (with 1½ tablespoons of low-calorie dressing). This adds about 70 Calories to the meal. Then the total for this dish would be 340 Calories.

Spaghetti Squash & Cheese

1½-pound spaghetti squash
2 cups grape tomatoes
4 teaspoons olive oil
2 teaspoons minced garlic
4 teaspoons bread crumbs
1¾ cups 2% milk
½ teaspoon kosher salt
½ teaspoon freshly ground black pepper
3 ounces part-skim mozzarella cheese, shredded (about ¾ cup)
1½ ounces Parmesan cheese, grated (about ⅓ cup)
½ cup torn fresh basil leaves

1. Preheat oven to 350°F. Halve the spaghetti squash and deseed. Place both halves in a in a casserole dish (cut-side down) filled with half cup water. Cook about 45 minutes. Allow to cool 10 minutes and then scrape out spaghetti flesh with a fork into a bowl.
2. Preheat broiler to high. Combine tomatoes and 2 teaspoons of oil in a jellyroll pan. Broil 3 minutes or until tomatoes begin to break down.
3. Place a small saucepan over medium heat. Add remaining 2 teaspoons oil to pan; swirl. Add garlic; cook 1 minute, stirring frequently. Stir in flour. Add milk, salt, and black pepper, stirring with a whisk. Bring to a simmer; cook 1 minute or until thickened, stirring frequently. Remove pan from heat; stir in all but 3 tablespoons of cheeses.
4. Stir cheese mixture into the spaghetti squash then place in a small 2 quart baking dish. Stir in tomato mixture and torn basil. Sprinkle remaining cheeses over spaghetti squash mixture. Broil 2 minutes or until the top is browned. Garnish with basil leaves.

Serves 6.   About 300 Calories per serving.

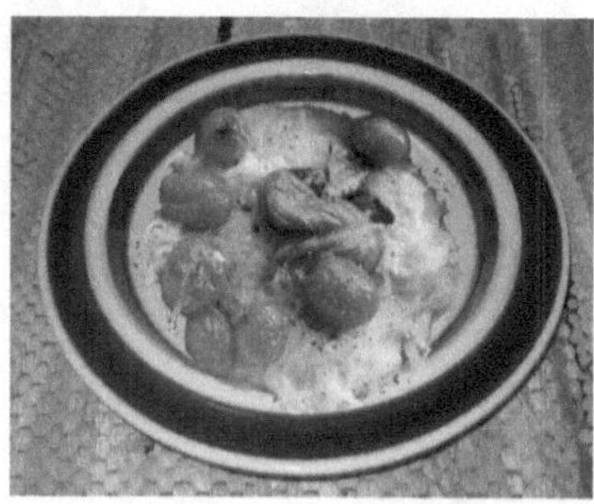

Note: Suggest this be served with ½ cup cooked brown rice and one cup steamed broccoli. This adds 150 Calories. Then the total for this meal would be 450 Calories.

Recipe 8

<u>Vegetarian Hash</u>

3 cups diced peeled sweet potato
2 tablespoons chopped fresh oregano
2 tablespoons olive oil
¾ teaspoon kosher salt, divided
½ teaspoon ground cumin
½ teaspoon ground cinnamon
¼ teaspoon ground red pepper
4 garlic cloves, minced
1¼ cups water, divided
1 cup green beans, trimmed and cut into 1-inch pieces
1 tablespoon adobo sauce
1 (15.5-ounce) can unsalted black beans, rinsed and drained
2 ounces soft white cheese, crumbled (about ½ cup)
¼ cup unsalted pumpkinseed kernels
1 plum tomato, seeded and diced

1. Heat a large skillet over medium-high heat. Add oil to pan; swirl. Add potato, oregano, and ½ teaspoon salt; cook 3 minutes, stirring occasionally. Add cumin, cinnamon, red pepper, and garlic; cook 1 minute.
2. Add ½ cup water; cover, reduce heat, and cook 5 minutes. Uncover; cook 2 minutes. Remove pan from heat.
3. Bring remaining ¾ cup water to a boil in a saucepan. Add remaining ¼ teaspoon salt and green beans; cook 4 minutes. Stir in adobo sauce and black beans.
4. Place ½ cup potato mixture in each of 4 shallow bowls; top each with ½ cup bean mixture, 2 tablespoons cheese, 1 tablespoon pumpkinseeds, and 1 tablespoon tomato.

<u>Serves 4.</u> About 320 Calories per serving

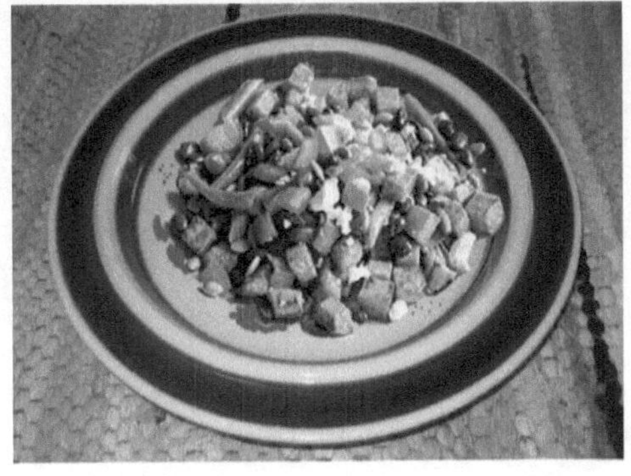

Recipe 9

<u>Portobello Mushroom Burger</u>

   ¼ cup low-sodium soy sauce
   ¼ cup balsamic vinegar
   2 tablespoons olive oil
   3 garlic cloves, minced
   4 (4-inch) portobello mushroom caps
   1 small red bell pepper
   ¼ cup light mayonnaise
   ½ teaspoon olive oil
   ⅛ teaspoon ground red pepper
   4 (2-ounce) hamburger buns
   4 (¼-inch-thick) slices tomato
   4 curly leaf lettuce leaves

1. Combine first 4 ingredients in a large zip-top plastic bag; add mushrooms to bag. Seal and marinate at room temperature for 2 hours, turning bag occasionally. Remove mushrooms from bag. Start grill to medium heat.
3. Cut bell pepper in half lengthwise; discard seeds and membranes. Place pepper halves on grill rack coated with cooking spray; grill 15 minutes or until blackened, turning occasionally. Place in a zip-top plastic bag; seal. Let stand 10 minutes. Peel. Finely chop 1 pepper half; place in a small bowl. Add mayonnaise, ½ teaspoon oil, and ground red pepper; stir well.
4. Place mushrooms, gill sides down, on grill rack coated with cooking spray; grill 4 minutes on each side. Place buns, cut sides down, on grill rack coated with cooking spray; grill 30 seconds on each side or until toasted. Spread 2 tablespoons mayonnaise mixture on top half of each bun. Place 1 mushroom on bottom half of each bun. Top each mushroom with 1 tomato slice and 1 lettuce leaf.

<u>Serves 4</u>. About 270 Calories per serving.

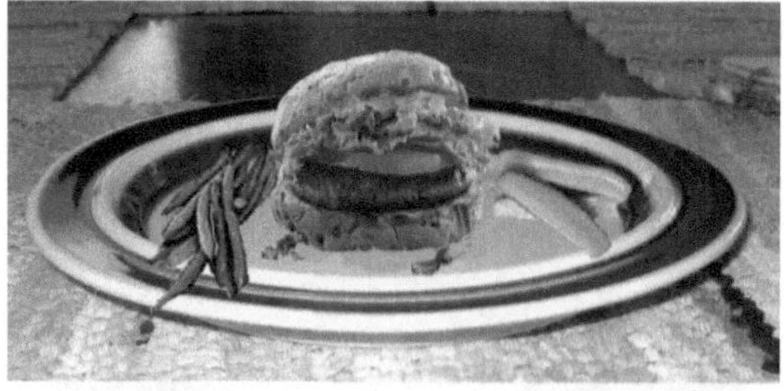

Note: The steamed green beans and pickles only add another 30 Calories - bringing the total for this meal up to 300 Calories.

<u>Hearty Vegetable Soup</u>

     2 15-oz cans white kidney beans, drained
     1 tablespoon olive oil
     ½ large yellow onion, chopped
     2 garlic cloves, minced
     1 cup chopped fresh tomatoes
     2 celery stalks, cut into ½-inch pieces
     1½ carrots, cut into ½-inch pieces
     5 cups vegetable stock
     1 medium potato, in ½-inch pieces
     ¼ cup chopped fresh basil
     ¼ head of red cabbage, in ½-inch pieces
     2 zucchini (summer squash) in ½-inch pieces

Heat olive oil in a large pot over medium heat. Add onion and garlic. Sauté 5 minutes. Add green cabbage, tomatoes, celery, and carrots. Sauté 10 minutes. Add beans, 5 cups of stock, potatoes, and basil. Bring to a boil. Reduce heat, cover and simmer for one hour. Add red cabbage, zucchini and salt. Cover and simmer until vegetables are tender, about 20 minutes longer. Stir in about ¼ cup Parmesan cheese.
<u>**Serves 4**</u>. 360 Calories per serving

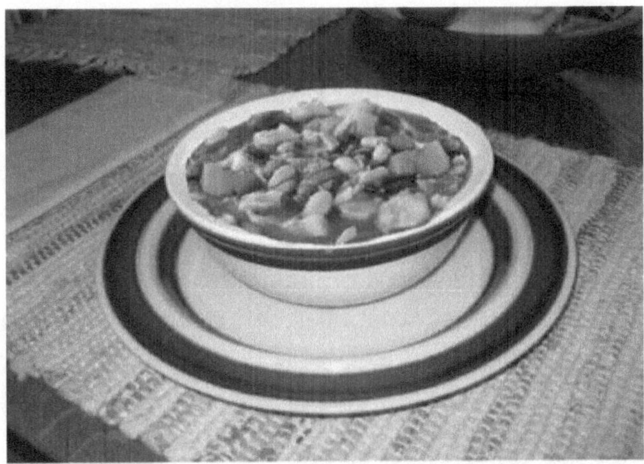

Note: Serve the vegetable soup with a small whole-grain roll. This adds about 80 Calories. Then the total for this meal would be 440 Calories.

Recipe 11

<u>Risotto Primavera</u>

 5 cups low-sodium vegetable broth
 3 tablespoons olive oil, divided
 3 tablespoons butter, divided
 ½ large yellow onion, finely diced
 3 carrots, finely diced
 1 cup cauliflower and broccoli pieces
 1 yellow squash, diced
 1½ cups Arborio rice
 1½ cups white wine
 4 green onions, thinly sliced
 ½ cup frozen peas
 4 ounces goat cheese
 ½ cup grated Parmesan cheese

1. Pour vegetable broth into a small saucepan. Heat to a simmer.

2. In large Dutch oven, heat 2 tablespoons olive oil and 2 tablespoons butter. Add diced onions and carrots. Stir and cook for about 1 minute. Add cauliflower and cook for another minute. Add broccoli and cook for 30 seconds. Then add squash and cook for 30 seconds. Sprinkle in salt and stir. Remove from Dutch oven and put on a plate. Set aside.

3. Add 1 tablespoon olive oil and 1 tablespoon butter to the Dutch oven. Over medium-low heat, add rice and stir, cooking for 1 minute. Add half the wine and 1½ teaspoons kosher salt. Stir and cook until liquid is absorbed. Over the next 30 to 45 minutes, add 1 cup of simmering vegetable broth from the small saucepan at a time, stirring and cooking until each addition of broth has been absorbed. Add other half cup of wine and cook until absorbed. Add green onions and peas, stirring to combine. Taste to make sure rice is the right texture; add more broth if rice has too much bite.

4. Once rice is cooked, remove from heat. Stir in goat cheese, Parmesan cheese, and vegetables until all goat cheese is combined. Serve on a plate with a sprig of dill.

<u>**Serves 8.**</u> About 365 Calories per serving

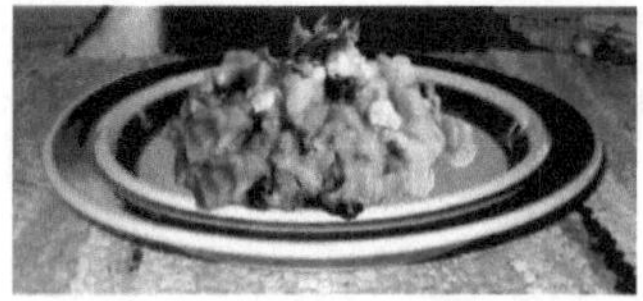

Note: Serve with a small whole-grain which brings the total for the meal to 445 Calories.

Recipe 12

<u>Vegetables with Couscous</u>

1 10-ounce box couscous
1 red bell pepper, cut into strips
1 yellow bell pepper, cut into strips
1 small yellow squash, sliced
1 small zucchini, sliced
1 teaspoon salt
¾ teaspoon black pepper
¾ teaspoon minced garlic
¾ teaspoon Italian seasoning
2 tablespoon olive oil
3 tablespoon balsamic vinegar
5 ounces feta cheese

1. Pre-heat oven to 425 ºF.
2. Prepare couscous according to package directions.
3. In a small bowl, whisk together marinade of salt, pepper, garlic, Italian seasoning, olive oil and balsamic vinegar and toss with pepper strips, sliced squash and zucchini.
4. Spread vegetables evenly in sheet pan and roast for 10 to 12 minutes or until vegetables are crisp-tender. Reserve left over marinade.
5. Allow vegetables to cool slightly, then toss with remaining marinade, couscous and feta cheese.

<u>Serves 6</u>. About 330 Calories per serving

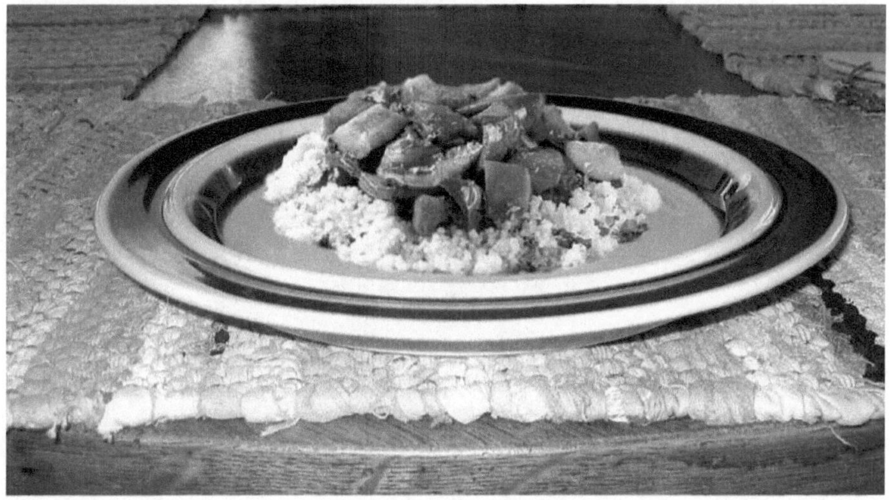

Note: Add a small whole-grain roll which brings the total for the meal to 410 Calories per serving.

Recipe 13

<u>Curried Eggplant & Tomato</u>

1	cup white basmati rice
1	tablespoon olive oil
1	onion, chopped
2	pints cherry tomatoes, halved
1	eggplant (about 1 pound), cut in ½-inch pieces
1	15.5-ounce can chickpeas, rinsed
1½	teaspoons curry powder
½	cup fresh basil

1) In medium saucepan with a tight-fitting lid, combine rice, 1½ cups water, and ½ teaspoon salt and bring to a boil. Stir rice once, cover, and reduce heat to low. Simmer for about 18 minutes. Remove from heat and let stand, covered, for 5 minutes.

2) Meanwhile, cook oil in saucepan over medium-high heat. Add onion and cook, stirring occasionally, until softened, 4 to 6 minutes.

3) Stir in tomatoes, eggplant, curry powder, 1 teaspoon salt, and ¼ teaspoon black pepper. Cook, stirring, until fragrant, about 2 minutes.

4) Add 2 cups water and bring to a boil. Reduce heat and simmer, partially covered, until eggplant is tender, about 12 to 15 minutes. Stir in chickpeas and cook until heated through, about 3 minutes.

5) Remove vegetables from heat and stir in basil. Fluff rice with a fork. Serve vegetables over steamed white rice.

<u>Serves 4</u>. About 325 Calories per serving (including rice).

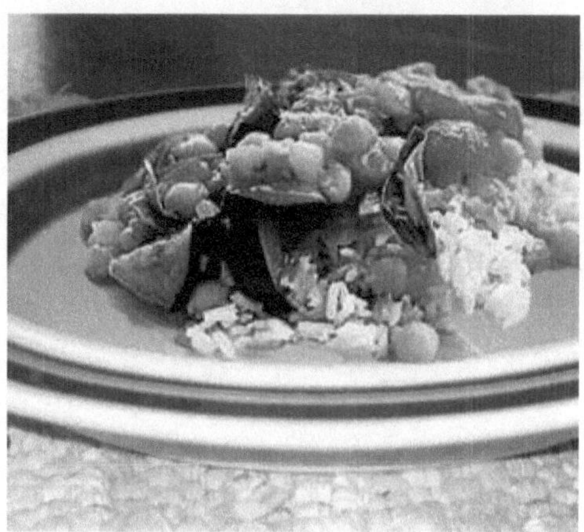

Note: Add a large tossed salad with 1½ tablespoons of low-cal dressing. This increases the calorie total to 395 per serving.

"""

<h1 style="text-align:center">Recipe 14</h1>

<u>Indian Shahi Paneer</u>

2 tablespoons cooking oil
1 large onion, thinly sliced
4 cloves garlic, minced
1 teaspoon ground cumin
1 teaspoon ground coriander
½ teaspoon ground turmeric
½ teaspoon red chili powder
4 tomatoes, pureed
½ pound paneer, cubed
1 teaspoon sugar
¼ cup cream
2 tablespoons chopped fresh cilantro

1) Cook oil in a large skillet over medium heat. Add onion and garlic in the hot oil until the onions are soft and golden brown, about 5 minutes. Sprinkle in cumin, coriander, turmeric, and chili powder over onion and garlic. Continue cooking until seasonings are fragrant, about 30 seconds.

2) Pour pureed tomatoes into skillet. Cook until excess liquid evaporates and oil separates, 3 to 5 minutes. Add paneer, ¼ cup water, sugar, and salt to mixture. Stir gently so paneer does not break apart. Cook until paneer begins to absorb some of liquid, about 10 minutes.

3) Stir cream into mixture and simmer another 5 minutes. Salt to taste. Serve with garnish of cilantro and steamed brown rice.

<u>Serves 4</u>. About 300 Calories per serving .

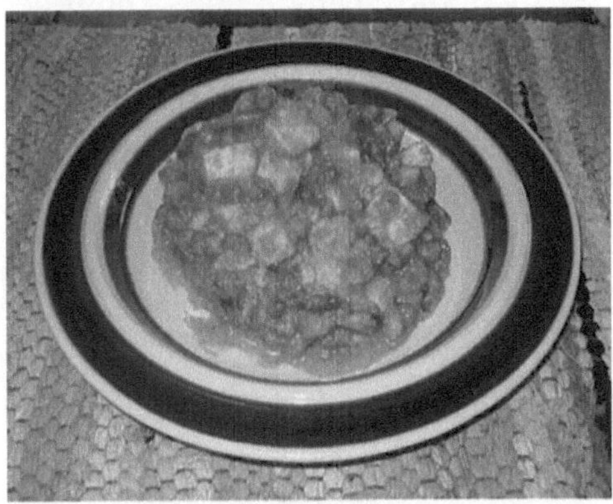

Note: We suggest you add ¼ cup of cooked brown rice and a large tossed salad (with 1½ tablespoons of low-calorie dressing). This adds about 120 Calories to the meal. Then the total for this dish would be 420 Calories per serving.

Recipe 15

<u>Soba Noodles & Broccoli Rabe</u>

    6 ounces soba noodles
    1 pound broccoli rabe
    2 tablespoons extra-virgin olive oil
    ½ teaspoon sesame seeds
    handful fresh cilantro, chopped

Peanut sauce:

    ½ cup peanut butter
    ¼ cup reduced sodium soy sauce
    3 tablespoons rice vinegar
    2 tablespoons honey
    1 teaspoon grated fresh ginger
    2 cloves garlic, pressed or minced
    ¼ teaspoon red pepper flakes

1) Prepare broccoli rabe by rinsing well and patting dry. Slice off tough lower stem ends.

2) Prepare peanut sauce: In 2-cup liquid measuring cup, whisk ingredients together with 3 tablespoons water. Set aside.

3) Bring large pot of salted water to boil. Meanwhile, warm 2 tablespoons olive oil in a large skillet over medium heat. Add broccoli rabe and season with a dash of salt and a small pinch of red pepper flakes. Toss to combine and continue cooking, stirring occasionally, until leaves have wilted and stems are easily pierced by a fork, about 8 minutes. Remove from heat.

4) Once water is boiling, add soba noodles and cook until al dente, about 5 minutes. Drain noodles and return them to pot. Add broccoli rabe and toss with peanut sauce.

5) Top individual servings with a sprinkle of chopped cilantro and sesame seeds.

<u>Serves 4</u>. About 490 Calories per serving

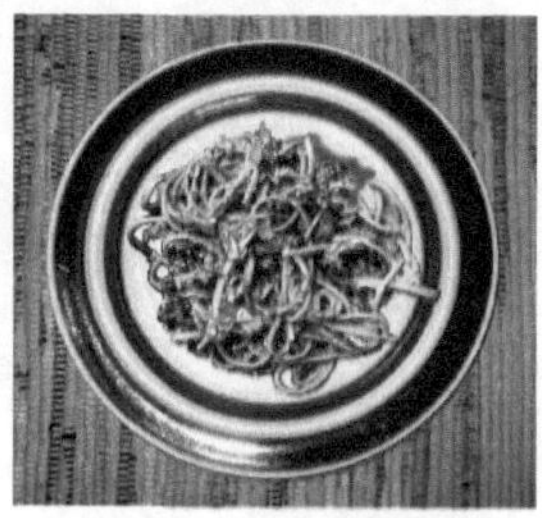

Note: Add a large tossed salad (with 1½ tablespoons of low-calorie dressing). Then the total for this meal would be 560 Calories per serving.

Recipe 16

<u>Healthy Frittata</u>

    3 large eggs, plus 3 egg whites
    ¾ cup reduced-fat cottage cheese
    4 ounces smoked gouda cheese, shredded (about 1 cup)
    1 teaspoon minced fresh rosemary
    3 cloves garlic, thinly sliced
    2 tablespoons olive oil
    1 medium onion, chopped
    16-ounce package frozen mixed vegetables, thawed
    2 tablespoons grated parmesan cheese
    1 scant teaspoon paprika

Position a rack in the upper third of your oven and preheat to 450 degrees F. Whisk eggs and egg whites in a bowl. Add the cottage cheese and whisk until almost smooth. Whisk in the gouda and rosemary. In a 10-inch nonstick skillet over medium-high, cook the garlic in the olive oil. Heat until garlic starts to brown, about 1 to 2 minutes. Add onion, season with salt and cook 2 minutes. Add the vegetables, increase the heat to high and cook until just tender, about 5 minutes. Reduce the heat to medium.

Spread the egg mixture evenly in the pan. Cook, without disturbing until a thin crust forms on the bottom, about 2 minutes. Run a rubber spatula around the edge to release egg from the pan. Continue cooking until the bottom is golden, about 2 to 3 minutes. Sprinkle with the parmesan and paprika. Transfer skillet to the oven and bake about 5 to 7 minutes. Remove from the oven, cover and let sit, 5 to 7 minutes. Cut into 4 wedges.
<u>Serves 4</u>. 320 Calories per serving (¼ of frittata)

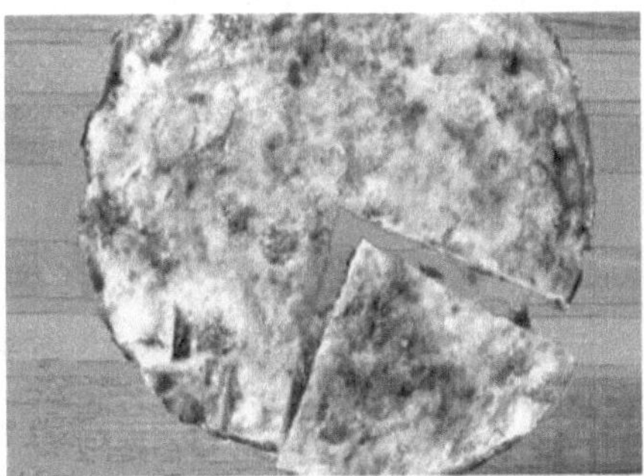

Photo shows frittata on cutting board - hot from skillet.

Note: Serve with a large tossed salad (with 1½ tablespoons of low-calorie dressing) and a small whole-grain roll. Then the total for this meal is 470 Calories.

Recipe 17

<u>Middle East Koshari</u>

This is the national dish of Egypt and a popular street food.

- 6 ounces uncooked noodles, cut to 1" pieces
- 1 tablespoon vegetable oil
- 1 cup uncooked white rice
- ½ cup lentils
- 2 onions, minced
- 1 clove garlic, minced
- 1½ tablespoons white vinegar
- 2 tomatoes (ripe), diced
- ¼ cup tomato paste
- 1 teaspoon ground cumin
- 1 15-ounce can chickpeas

1) Cook pasta according to package directions. Drain, cover and keep warm.

2) Heat ½ tablespoon vegetable oil in saucepan over medium-high heat. Stir in rice until it is coated with oil, about 3 minutes. Add 1½ cups water and ½ teaspoon salt. Bring to boil; reduce heat to low, cover and simmer until rice is tender and liquid is absorbed, 20 to 25 minutes.

3) Soak lentils for 30 minutes. Drain and rinse. Cook according to package directions.

4) Heat ½ tablespoon vegetable oil in a large skillet over medium-high heat. Add onions stirring often until they begin to brown, 10 to 15 minutes. Add garlic and cook another minute. Remove from pan, drain on a paper towel-lined plate.

5) Place half onion mixture in saucepan. Mix in vinegar. Add chopped tomatoes and tomato paste, black pepper, 1 teaspoon salt and cumin. Bring to boil then reduce heat to medium-low and simmer about 12 minutes. Add chickpeas and cook another minute.

6) Serve by placing a spoonful of rice, then macaroni, and then lentils on serving plates. Sprinkle with some browned onions. Top with tomato sauce and chickpeas.

<u>Serves 6</u>. About 370 Calories per serving.

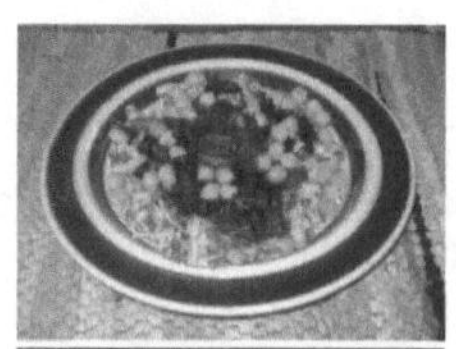

Note: We suggest this dish be accompanied by a large tossed salad with 1½ tablespoons of low-cal dressing. Then the total for the meal is 440 Calories.

Recipe 18

<u>Veggie & Egg Fried Rice</u>

    6 teaspoons soy sauce
    1 teaspoon sesame oil
    1 tablespoon Canola oil
    2 large eggs, beaten
    1 cup diced onion
    1 cup diced carrots
    8 oz mushrooms, sliced
    1/2 cup frozen peas
    4 cups cooked jasmine rice
    3 green onions, sliced

1. In a small bowl whisk together soy sauce and sesame oil and set aside.
2. Heat 1 teaspoon canola oil in a large skillet over medium high heat. Add eggs and scramble until cooked through. Remove from pan and set aside.
3. Heat remaining oil in pan over medium high heat. Add onions, carrots and mushrooms. Cook, stirring occasionally, until veggies are soft, about 5 minutes.
4. Add peas to pan and cook for about one minute, or until soft. Stir in cooked jasmine rice into pan breaking up any large lumps of rice. Add cooked eggs back to pan.
5. Pour soy sauce and sesame oil mixture into pan and stir until ingredients are completely coated. Heat through (about 2 minutes). Mix in green onions.

<u>Serves 4.</u> About 360 Calories per serving.

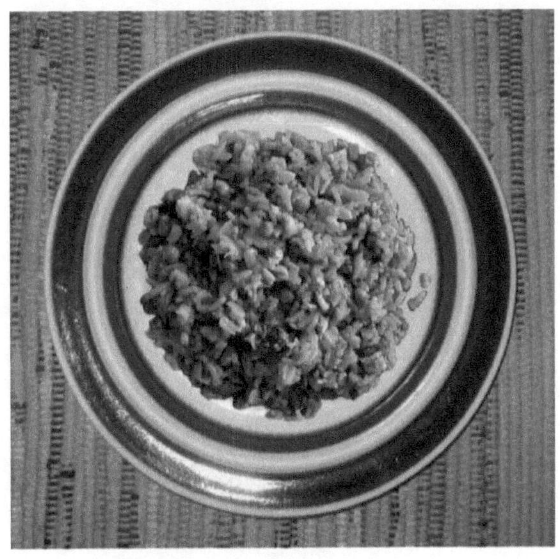

Recipe 19

Sweet & Sour Lentils over Rice

    1 cup dry lentils 3 tablespoons seasoned rice vinegar
    3 tablespoons low-sodium soy sauce
    3 tablespoons ketchup
    ½ teaspoon ground ginger
    2 teaspoons brown sugar
    8 oz can pineapple chunks in natural juice, reserve juice
    1 red bell pepper, sliced
    1 green bell pepper, sliced
    ¼ yellow onion, sliced
    1 tablespoon cornstarch
    2 cups cooked brown rice

1) Cook lentils according to package directions. Set aside.

2) Sweet & Sour Sauce: Combine vinegar, soy sauce, ketchup, ginger, brown sugar and pineapple juice in small bowl. Whisk until well-combined. Set sauce aside.

3) To a large skillet, add thin layer of water. Heat until very hot. Lower heat to medium and add peppers and onions to pan. Cook for 8 to 10 minutes, or until softened. Add more water, if needed.

4) Add cooked lentils and pineapple to the skillet. Stir until well-combined.

5) In small bowl, add 1 tablespoon cornstarch to 2 tablespoons cold water. Mix well.

6) Lower the heat to medium-low and add sweet and sour sauce mixture. Stir in cornstarch-water mixture to thicken sauce. Continue simmering the lentil mixture for 3 to 5 minutes, or until the sauce has thickened to your liking. Add additional cornstarch and water if desired.

7) Serve over warm cooked rice.

Serves 4. About 460 Calories per serving.

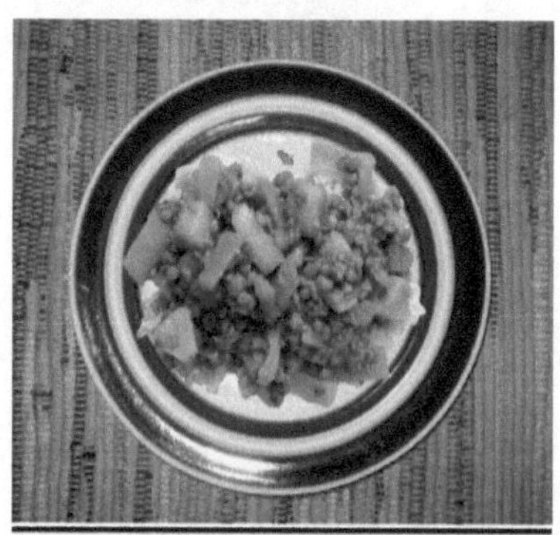

<u>Tofu Steak with Veggies</u>

⅓ cup white miso (soybean paste)
⅓ cup mirin (sweet rice wine)
⅓ cup rice vinegar
1 tablespoon finely grated peeled fresh ginger
½ cup chopped dry-roasted peanuts, divided
5 tablespoons sesame oil, divided
2 (14-ounce) packages water-packed firm tofu, drained
8 cups salad greens

1. Combine white miso, mirin, ¼ cup peanuts, and 3 tablespoons oil in a small bowl; stir with a whisk.
2. Cut each tofu block crosswise into 8 (½-inch-thick) slices. Arrange tofu on several layers of paper towels. Top with several more layers of paper towels; top with a cast-iron skillet or other heavy pan. Let stand 30 minutes. Remove tofu from paper towels.
3. Heat 1 tablespoon oil in a large nonstick skillet over medium-high heat. Add 4 tofu slices to pan; sauté 4 minutes on each side or until crisp and golden. Remove from pan, and drain tofu on paper towels. Repeat procedure with remaining 1 tablespoon oil and remaining 4 tofu slices.
4. Place 1 cup greens on each of 8 plates. Top each serving with 2 tofu slices, 3 tablespoons miso mixture, and 1½ teaspoons chopped peanuts.

<u>**Serves 8**</u>: About 275 Calories per serving.

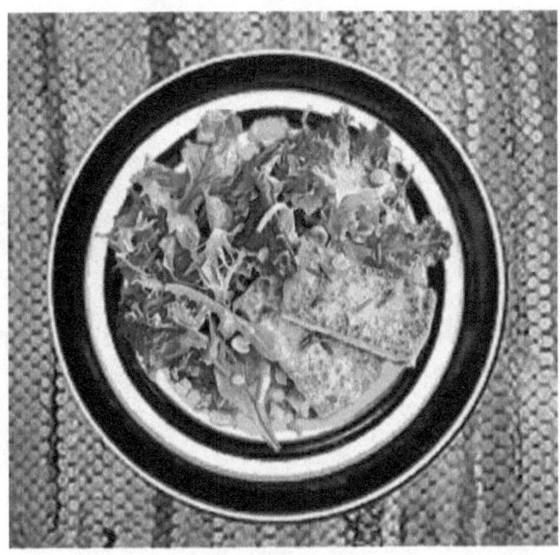

Note: Add a small whole-grain which brings the total for the meal to 355 Calories.

Recipe 21

<u>Tofu, Bok Choy & Mushroom Stir Fry</u>

2 (14-ounce) packages water-packed firm tofu, drained
2 tablespoons sesame oil
3 cloves minced garlic
½ cup sliced shiitake mushrooms
½ cup sliced button mushrooms
2 teaspoons canola oil
1 tablespoon soy sauce
1 bok choy, chopped (or 2 to 3 baby bok choy)
6 scallions (green onions), sliced
¼ cup vegetable broth
2 teaspoons fresh ginger, grated
2 teaspoons sesame oil

1) Go to Appendix A (page 109) for instructions re preparation of tofu steaks. (Cut each tofu block crosswise into 8 (½-inch-thick) slices.)
2) Sauté garlic and mushrooms in canola oil for 3 to 5 minutes. Add in soy sauce, bok choy and scallions, and cook for about 3 more minutes.
3) Reduce heat to medium low and add vegetable broth and ginger. Simmer for another 3 to 5 minutes.
4) Stir in the sesame oil and remove from heat.
5) Serve bok choy and mushroom stir-fry with 2 tofu steaks over brown rice.

<u>Serves 4.</u> About 430 Calories per serving (including tofu and ½ cup brown rice).

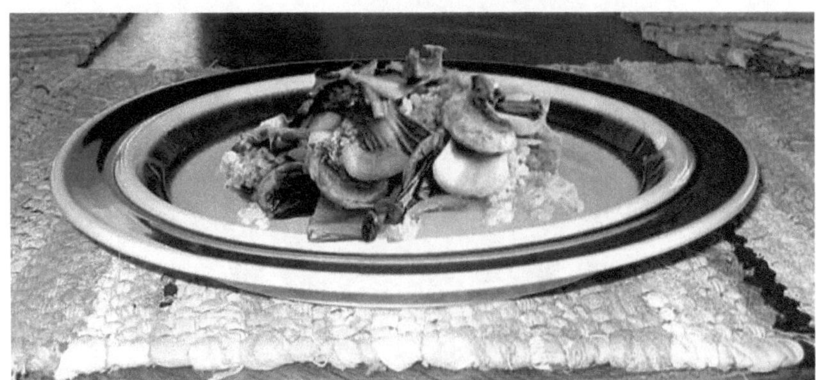

Tofu steaks not shown in photo.

Note: Add a small whole-grain roll which brings the total for the meal to 510 Calories.

Recipe 22

<u>Tofu & Broccoli in Garlic Sauce</u>

    1 medium onion, diced
    4 cloves garlic, minced
    3 tablespoon olive oil
    2 cups broccoli, chopped
    1 (14-ounce) package water-packed firm tofu, drained
    1½ teaspoons ginger powder
    ¼ teaspoon cayenne pepper
    3 tablespoon corn starch
    ¼ cup soy sauce
    1 cup water

1. Go to Appendix A (page 109) for Tofu preparation instructions. (Cut tofu into 1-inch cubes.)
2. In a large skillet, over medium heat, sauté onions and garlic in olive oil until onions turn clear, about 3-5 minutes.
3. Add the tofu, ginger, cayenne and broccoli to the pan and continue to cook until broccoli is done, another 6-8 minutes.
4. In a separate small bowl, mix together the corn starch, soy sauce and water. Then add this mixture to the broccoli and tofu. Cook until sauce thickens, then remove from heat.
5. Serve over brown rice.

<u>**Serves 4**</u>. About 320 Calories per serving (not including rice).

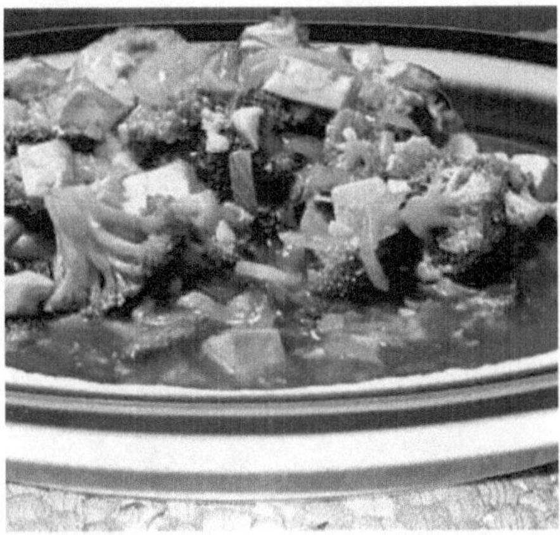

Note: We suggest you add ½ cup of cooked brown rice and a large tossed salad (with 1½ tablespoons of low-calorie dressing). This adds about 170 Calories to the meal. Then the total for this dish would be 490 Calories per serving.

Recipe 23

<u>Tofu Szechuan Style</u>

   1 14-ounce packages firm tofu, packed in water
   ½ cup less-sodium chicken broth
   1 tablespoon sambal oelek (chili paste)
   1 tablespoon less-sodium soy sauce
   1 teaspoon cornstarch
   2 teaspoons black bean garlic sauce
   1 tablespoon canola oil
   1 (8-ounce) package pre-sliced mushrooms
   ½ cup matchstick-cut carrots
   1 tablespoon ground fresh ginger
   ½ cup chopped green onions
   ¼ cup unsalted dry-roasted peanuts, chopped

1) Go to Appendix A (page 109) for Tofu preparation instructions. (After draining, cut tofu into 1-inch cubes.)

2) Arrange tofu in a single layer on a foil-lined jelly-roll pan coated with cooking spray; broil 14 minutes or until golden.

3) While tofu cooks, combine broth and next 4 ingredients (through black bean sauce), stirring with a whisk; set aside.

4) Heat oil in a large nonstick skillet over medium-high heat. Add salt and mushrooms; sauté 4 minutes or until mushrooms begin to release liquid, stirring occasionally. Stir in carrots and ginger; cook 1 minute. Add broth mixture; cook 30 seconds or until sauce begins to thicken. Remove from heat; stir in tofu and onions. Serve over rice; sprinkle with peanuts.

<u>Serves 4</u>. About 410 Calories per serving (including rice).

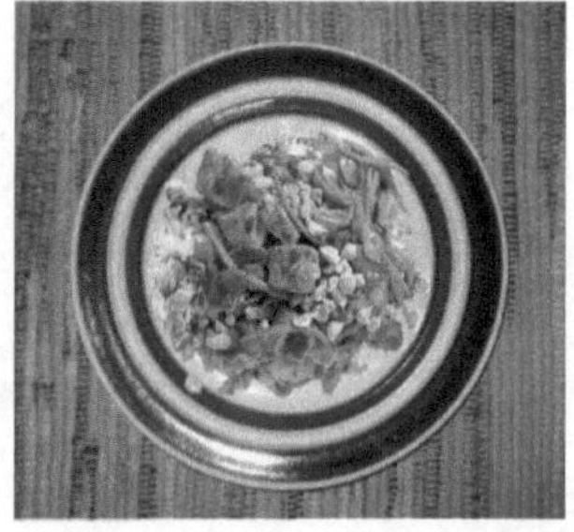

Note: We suggest you add a large tossed salad (with 1½ tablespoons of low-calorie dressing). Then the total for this dish would be 480 Calories per serving.

Recipe 24

<u>Asian Tofu with Veggies</u>

    1 14-ounce packages firm tofu, packed in water
    2 tablespoons olive oil, divided
    5 cups assorted stir-fry vegetables (see photo)
    ½ cup Chinese hot sauce, such as Sriracha*
    ½ cup sweet chili sauce, such as Thai Kitchen
    ¼ cup soy sauce

1. Go to Appendix A (page 109) for instruction on how to drain tofu. After draining, slice tofu into 1-inch cubes.
2. In a large skillet, over medium heat, sauté vegetables in olive oil until vegetables are cooked through, about 3-5 minutes. In the same skillet, heat the other tablespoon of olive oil over medium heat and brown tofu on both sides, 4-5 minutes.
3. While the tofu is cooking, combine the hot sauce, sweet chili sauce and soy sauce in a small bowl.
4. For each serving, place the tofu and vegetables over ½ cup brown rice and top with sauce.

<u>Serves 4.</u> 370 Calories per serving

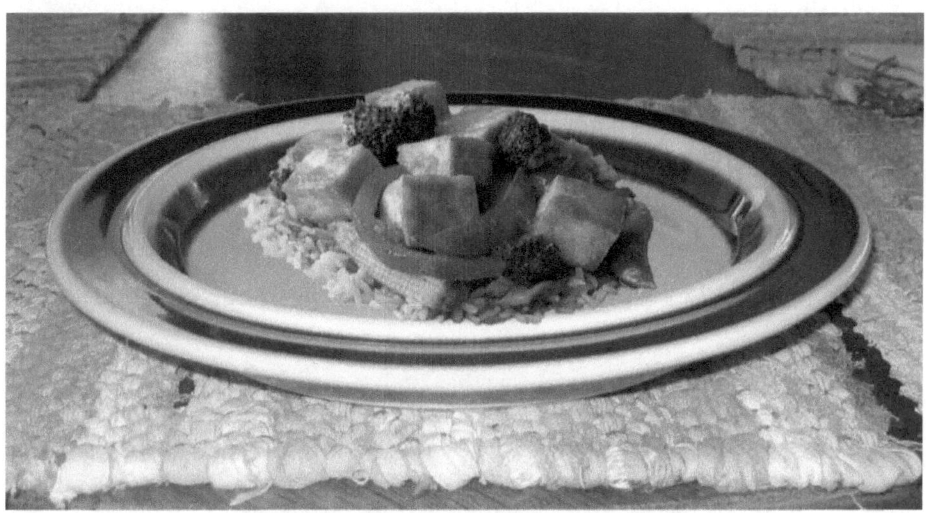

* Sriracha, is a Chinese hot sauce produced by Huy Fong Inc.

Recipe 25

<u>Cashew Tofu Stir Fry</u>

3 cloves garlic, minced
1 teaspoon fresh ginger, minced
2 tablespoons peanut oil
8 ounces extra-firm tofu, pressed
¾ cup mushrooms, sliced
1 4-ounce can bamboo shoots, drained & sliced thin
2 stalks celery, sliced
1 large green bell pepper, chopped
⅓ cup vegetable broth
2 tablespoons soy sauce
1 tablespoon cornstarch mixed with 3 tablespoons water
½ cup cashews
3 green onions, chopped

1. For tofu draining and preparation tips click see Appendix A (page 109). Cut tofu into 1-inch cubes.

2. In a large skillet or wok, heat oil and add garlic and ginger for about 2 minutes. Then add the tofu, carefully stirring to mix up the ginger and garlic. Cook for 3 to 4 minutes, or until tofu is lightly golden.

3. Add bell pepper and celery, and cook, stirring for about a minute. Then add mushrooms and bamboo shoots.

4. Add vegetable broth and soy sauce. Allow to simmer for another minute or two, until vegetables are tender but not yet done.

5. Stir in water-cornstarch mixture, heat until thickened and vegetables are done. Then stir in cashews and green onions, to combine well. Serve over steamed white rice.

<u>Serves 4</u>. About 275 Calories per serving (including ½ cup cooked rice).

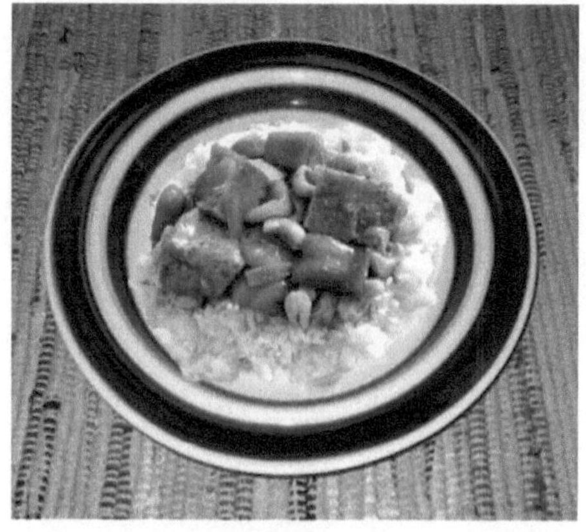

Tofu-Veggie Stir Fry

Citrus Sauce:
    6 tablespoons cooking wine
    ¼ cup orange juice
    1 tablespoon light soy sauce
    2 teaspoons toasted sesame oil
    1 teaspoon grated or minced fresh ginger
    1 teaspoon cornstarch
    1 tablespoon toasted sesame seeds
Stir Fry:
    1 (14-ounce) package firm tofu, drained
    1 tablespoon cooking oil
    1½ cups fresh or frozen sugar snap peas
    3 medium carrots, thinly sliced
    ¾ cup thinly sliced onion

1. Stir together sauce ingredients. Set aside while preparing stir fry.
2. Press and pat tofu dry with a towel to remove excess water. Cut into ½-inch cubes.
3. Heat a large skillet or wok over medium-high heat. Add oil and tofu; stir frequently until tofu is lightly browned, about 5 minutes. Add snow peas, carrots and onion. Stir-fry about 5 minutes until vegetables are cooked, but still crisp.
4. Stir in prepared sauce and cook 1-2 minutes until sauce is slightly thickened. Serve immediately.
Serves 4. 230 Calories per serving

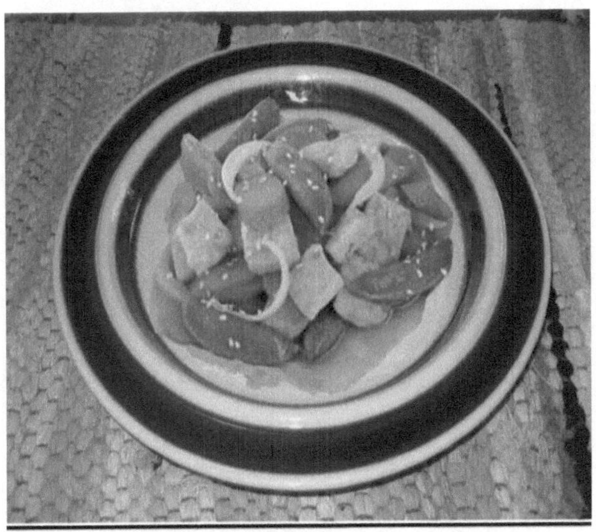

Recipe 27

<u>Teriyaki Tofu & Veggies</u>

    2 tablespoons sesame oil, divided
    3 cups broccoli florets
    2 cups zucchini, quartered & cut in ½ inch slices
    2 cups white button mushrooms, quartered
    1 cup carrots, sliced diagonally
    ½ medium red pepper, sliced
    1 block (14 oz) firm or extra-firm tofu, cubed

Teriyaki Sauce
    4 tablespoons soy sauce
    2 tablespoons sriracha (optional)
    3 cloves garlic, minced
    1 tablespoon brown sugar
    1 tablespoon peanut butter
    1½ tablespoons sesame oil

1) In a medium sized bowl, combine all of the teriyaki sauce ingredients.

2) Heat 1 tablespoon sesame oil in wok or skillet over medium-high heat. Arrange cubed tofu in wok. Cook both sides of tofu until golden-brown, about 3 to 4 minutes on each side. Once tofu is cooked, place in prepared teriyaki sauce and let sit while vegetables are cooked.

3) Heat 1 tablespoon sesame oil in a skillet or wok over medium-high heat. Add broccoli, toss, and cook for 2 minutes, stirring regularly. Add zucchini and carrots, toss, and cook for 3 minutes, stirring regularly. Add the mushroom and red pepper, toss, and cook for another 2-3 minutes until the broccoli is tender yet crisp. Add a few dashes of soy sauce and toss to coat. Put veggies in a bowl and set aside.

4) Reheat wok (or skillet) and put tofu and teriyaki sauce mixture into hot pan. Sauce should
bubble and thicken. Stir constantly to prevent burning. Remove from heat once sauce thickens, about 1 minute. Serve tofu and vegetables with ½ cup brown rice.

<u>Serves 4.</u> About 400 Calories per serving (including rice).

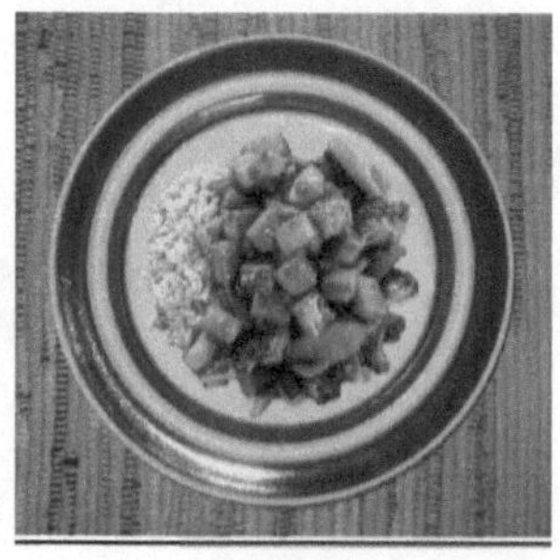

Crumbly-Tofu Scramble

16 ounces water-packed extra firm tofu
4 cups kale, chopped
3 tablespoons sesame oil
½ medium red onion, thinly sliced
1 medium red pepper, thinly sliced
1 teaspoon sea salt
1 teaspoon garlic powder
1 teaspoon cumin powder
½ teaspoon chili powder

For tofu draining and preparation tips see Appendix A (page 109). While tofu is draining, prepare sauce by adding garlic, cumin and chili powder to a small bowl and adding enough water to make a pourable sauce. Set aside.

Warm a large skillet over medium heat. Add 2 tablespoons sesame oil, onion and red pepper. Season with a pinch of salt and pepper and stir. Cook until softened - about 5 minutes. Add kale, season with a bit more salt and pepper, and cover to steam for about 2 minutes.

Meanwhile, unwrap tofu and use a fork to crumble into bite-sized pieces. Use a spatula to move the veggies to one side of the pan and add tofu. Sauté for 2 minutes, then add sauce, pouring it mostly over the tofu and a little over the veggies. Stir immediately, evenly distributing the sauce. Cook for another 5 to 7 minutes.

Serves 4. About 250 Calories per serving (not including potatoes).

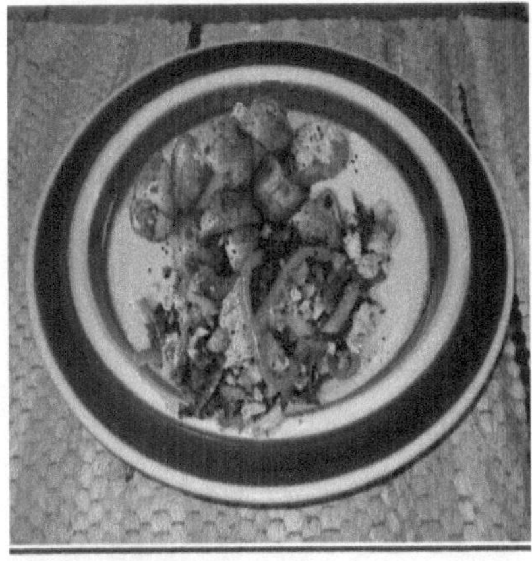

Note: Serve the tofu scramble with four small roasted potatoes and a large tossed salad (with 1½ tablespoons of low-calorie dressing). This adds about 150 Calories. Then the total for this meal, as shown, is 400 Calories

<u>Tofu with Veggies & Peanuts</u>

1 14-ounce package water-packed firm tofu
½ cup fat-free, less-sodium vegetable broth
1 tablespoon ground fresh chili paste
1 tablespoon less-sodium soy sauce
1 teaspoon cornstarch
2 teaspoons black bean garlic sauce
1 tablespoon canola oil
1 8-ounce package pre-sliced mushrooms
1 tablespoon bottled ground fresh ginger
½ cup matchstick-cut carrots
½ cup chopped green onions
¼ cup unsalted dry-roasted peanuts, chopped

1. Preheat broiler. Cook rice according to package directions, omitting salt and fat.
2. Drain tofu and cut into 1-inch pieces. (For tofu draining and preparation tips again see Appendix A (page 109)   Arrange tofu in a single layer on a foil-lined pan coated with cooking spray. Broil 14 minutes or until golden.
3. While tofu cooks, combine broth and next 4 ingredients (through black bean sauce), stirring with a whisk; set aside.
4. Heat oil in large nonstick skillet over medium-high heat. Add salt (to taste) and mushrooms; sauté 4 minutes or until mushrooms begin to release liquid, stirring occasionally. Stir in carrots and ginger; cook 1 minute. Add broth mixture; cook 30 seconds or until sauce thickens. Remove from heat; stir in tofu and onions. Serve over rice; sprinkle with peanuts.
<u>Serves 4</u>. About 320 Calories per serving

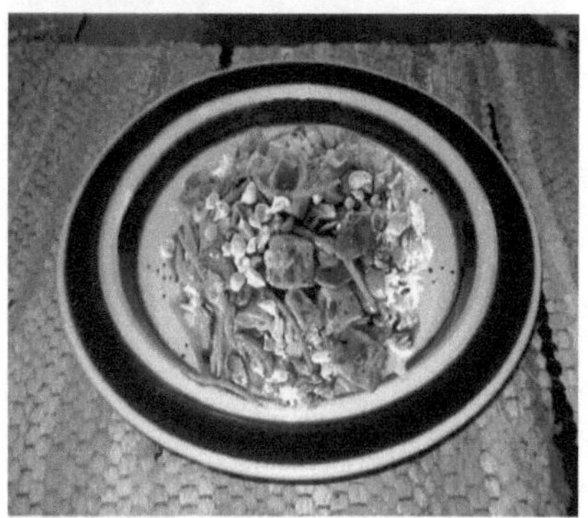

Note: Add a medium baked potato (no butter) and a small whole-grain roll. This increases the calorie total by 180. Then the meal would amount to 500 Calories.

Recipe 30

<u>Fried Tofu Salad</u>

1 14-ounce package water-packed firm tofu
½ cup cornstarch
1 cup Buffalo sauce*
⅛ cup sesame oil
8 cups chopped romaine lettuce
3 celery stalks, diced
2 plum tomatoes, diced
2 handfuls white corn tortilla chips, crumbled
½ cup low-calorie ranch dressing
½ cup bleu cheese crumbles

1. In large skillet heat ⅛ cup of oil over medium-high heat. Place tofu cubes in corn starch, evenly coating. Add tofu cubes to skillet. This may be done in 2 or 3 batches; do not over crowd tofu. Fry tofu for 2-3 minutes on each side, or until crispy. Use slotted spoon to remove tofu from oil and set on paper towels. Continue until all tofu is fried.
2. Place tofu in small bowl and toss with ⅓ cup of buffalo sauce until evenly coated. Set aside.
3. Distribute lettuce on four plates. Top each plate with celery, tomatoes, tortilla chips, ⅛ cup of bleu cheese crumbles. Add ¼ of tofu and pour ⅛ cup ranch dressing. Toss to combine.

<u>Serves 4.</u> About 450 Calories per serving.

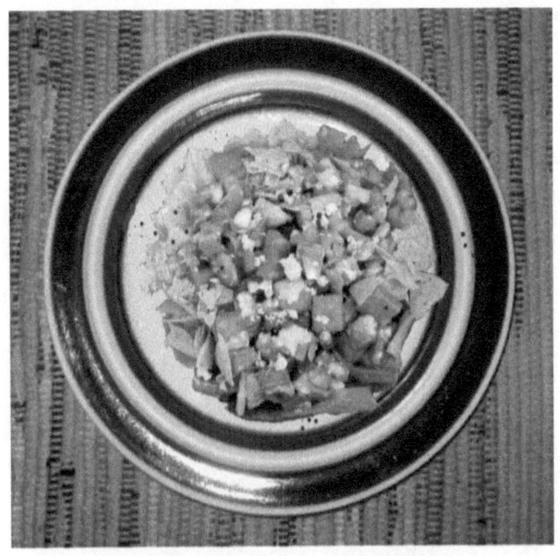

* Such as Frank's Buffalo Sauce. Can also use Sriracha, a Chinese hot sauce produced by Huy Fong Inc.

Recipe 31

Indian Crusted Tofu Salad

- 2 broccoli crowns
- 2 red bell peppers
- ½ teaspoon red pepper flakes
- 1 14-ounce package water-packed extra firm tofu
- ½ cup cornstarch
- ⅛ cup sesame oil
- 4 teaspoons sesame seeds, toasted
- 3 teaspoons ginger, minced
- 2 teaspoons garlic, minced
- 3 teaspoons chili sauce*
- 3 teaspoons soy sauce, lower sodium
- 3 teaspoons lime juice

1) Steam broccoli crowns for about 1 minute, or until tender. Set aside.

2) Press and cut tofu block into ½" cubes. Place tofu cubes in cornstarch to coat.

3) In a large skillet heat ⅛ cup oil over medium-high heat. Add tofu cubes to pot. This may be done in 2 or 3 batches; do not over crowd tofu. Fry tofu for 2-3 minutes on each side, or until crispy. Use slotted spoon to remove tofu from oil and set on paper towels. Continue until all tofu is fried.

4) Remove about half oil remaining in skillet, add broccoli, red pepper and red pepper flakes and toss in high heat for 1 minute. Remove ingredients and set aside.

5) In same skillet, add ginger and garlic. Cook for about 1 minute on medium heat. Add chili sauce, soy sauce and lime juice and cook to a boil.

6) Remove skillet from heat; add fried tofu, broccoli and red bell peppers and toss to coat. Top with toasted sesame seeds a serve as a hearty salad.

Serves 4. About 270 Calories per serving.

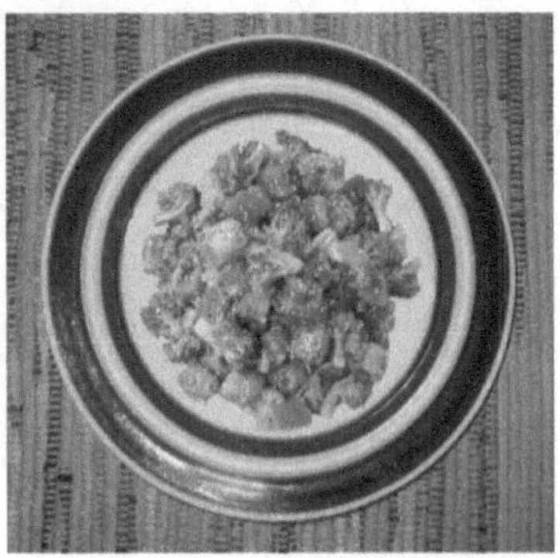

* Such as Sriracha sauce.

Recipe 32

<u>Tofu & Coconut Milk Curry</u>

2 cups cooked white rice
⅛ cup sesame oil
1 14-oz package firm tofu
½ cup cornstarch
2 broccoli crowns
2 bell peppers, chopped
1 yellow summer squash, sliced
2 tablespoons red curry paste
8 ounces canned coconut milk
Cilantro for garnish

1. Cook rice according to package directions.
2. Press and drain tofu and cut block into ½" cubes. Place tofu cubes in cornstarch to coat.
3. In a large skillet heat ⅛ cup oil over medium-high heat. Add tofu cubes to pot. This may be done in 2 or 3 batches; do not over crowd tofu. Fry tofu for 2-3 minutes on each side, or until crispy. Use slotted spoon to remove tofu from oil and set on paper towels. Continue until all tofu is fried.
4. Remove about half oil remaining in skillet, add broccoli, bell peppers, and squash. Cook over medium heat, stirring occasionally, about 3 minutes. Add curry paste and stir until vegetables are coated, then pour in coconut milk. Simmer until slightly thickened, about 10 minutes.
5. Divide tofu, rice and curry among four plates and garnish with cilantro.

<u>Serves 4</u>. About 460 Calories per serving.

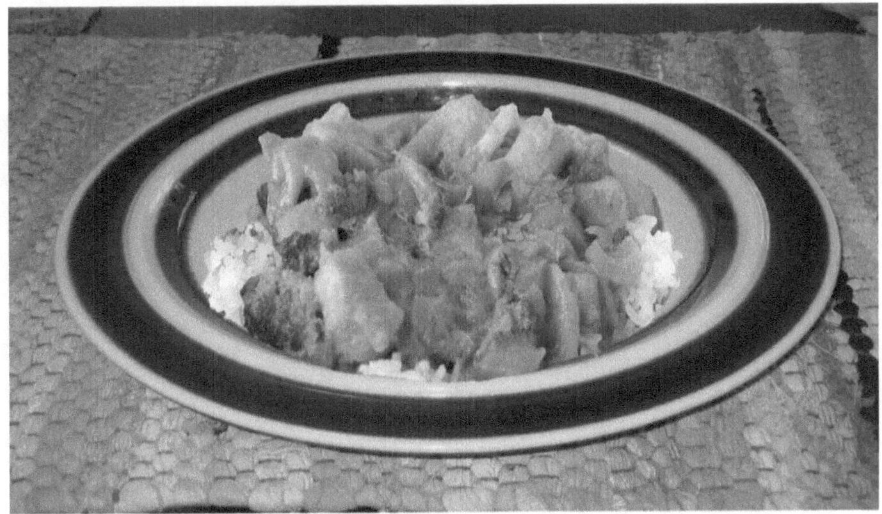

<h1 style="text-align:center">Recipe 33</h1>

<u>Tofu & Chinese Broccoli Stir Fry</u>

4 cloves garlic, minced 20
2 scallions, sliced 10
1 small piece ginger, minced
1 bunch Chinese broccoli, chopped 30
1 14-oz package firm tofu 365
¼ cup roasted peanuts, chopped 215
1 teaspoon Szechuan peppercorns 30
1 cup uncooked brown rice 735
2 tablespoons vinegar 20
2 tablespoons soy sauce 15
1½ tablespoons cornstarch 45
2 dried chili peppers
2 tablespoons sesame oil 225

1) Cook rice according to package directions.
2) Press and drain tofu and cut block into 1-inch cubes.
3) In a large skillet heat 2 tablespoons oil over medium-high heat. Add tofu cubes to pot. This may be done in 2 or 3 batches; do not over crowd tofu. Fry tofu for 2-3 minutes on each side, or until crispy. Use slotted spoon to remove tofu from oil and set on paper towels. Continue until all tofu is fried.
4) While tofu is cooking, make slurry: In small bowl, whisk together cornstarch, soy sauce, vinegar and ½ cup water.
5) In same skillet, heat two teaspoons of oil on medium-high until hot. Add Chinese broccoli and cook 1 to 2 minutes, or until bright green. Add scallions, ginger and garlic and cook about 1 minute, or until fragrant, stirring frequently.
6) In same skillet, stir in slurry, sesame oil, whole dried chiles and peppercorns. Cook for about 30 seconds, or until thoroughly combined. Stir in the browned tofu and cook another 1 to 2 minutes, or until sauce thickens; season with salt and pepper to taste.
7) Plate food and garnish with chopped peanuts.

<u>Serves 4</u>. About 430 Calories per serving.

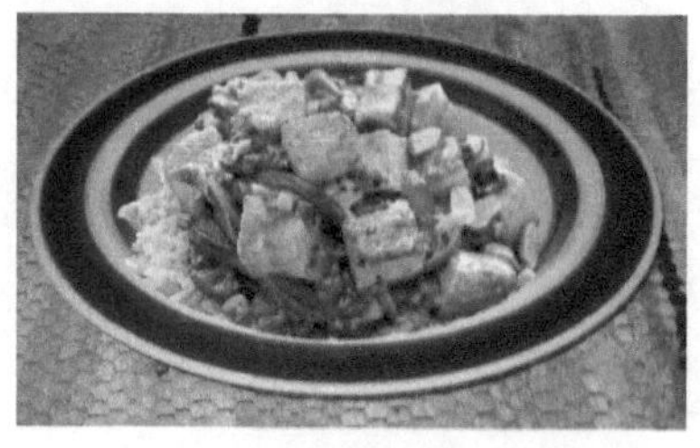

Recipe 34

<u>Tofu Scramble 2</u>

    1½ tablespoon sesame oil
    2   yellow onions, chopped
    3   cloves of garlic, minced
    1   tablespoon turmeric
    1½ packages firm tofu, drained and dried
    ½   cup sun-dried tomatoes
    1   small bunch basil leaves, torn

1) Heat oil in a large pan over medium high heat. When hot, add onions and garlic. Then cook until onions and garlic are soft, about 3 minutes.

2) Crumble tofu into the pan and add turmeric and ½ cup of water. Cook for an additional 3 to 5 minutes or until water has evaporated.

3) Take off heat and sprinkle in sun-dried tomatoes and basil leaves. Stir scramble and serve immediately.

<u>Serves 4.</u> About 260 Calories per serving.

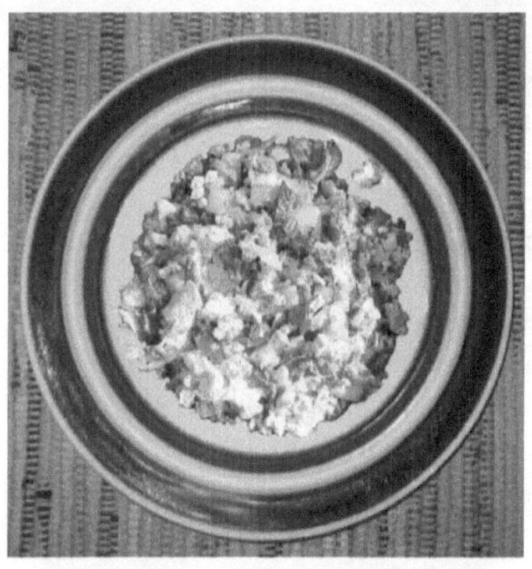

Recipe 35

Tofu with Noodles & Veggies

    1 12.3-oz. package extra-firm tofu, drained
    ½ cups low-sodium soy sauce
    3 tablespoons lime juice
    1 tablespoon rice vinegar
    2 teaspoons sesame oil
    2 teaspoons sugar
    1 tablespoon chopped fresh ginger
    1 clove garlic, chopped
    1 teaspoon Sriracha hot chili sauce
    8 ounces rice noodles
    3 carrots, shredded
    1 red bell pepper, thinly sliced
    8 scallions, thinly sliced
    1 8-oz. can diced water chestnuts, drained
    1 cup thinly sliced snow peas
    2 tablespoons sesame seeds

1) Drain and cut tofu into 1-inch cubes.

2) In a shallow bowl, whisk together soy sauce, lime juice, rice vinegar, sesame oil, sugar, ginger, garlic and chili sauce. Toss tofu in sauce and arrange in a single layer. Cover and chill for 15 minutes. Remove tofu, setting aside soy sauce mixture.

3) Cook noodles according to package directions. Drain and rinse noodles under cold water.

4) Combine noodles, reserved soy sauce mixture, carrots, bell pepper, scallions, water chestnuts and snow peas, tossing to coast. Add tofu; gently toss to combine. Fold in sesame seeds and serve.

Serves 4. About 310 Calories per serving.

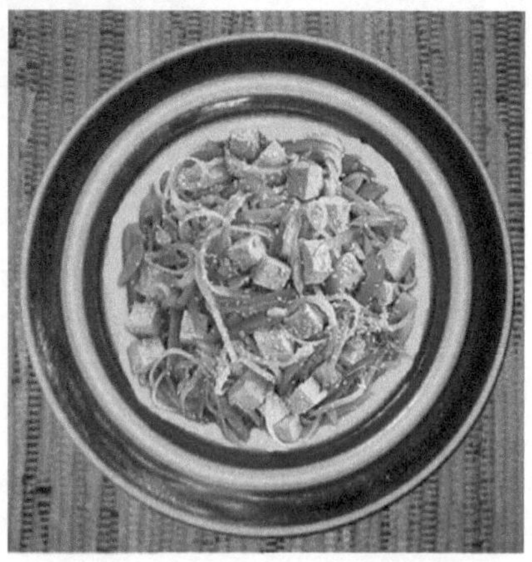

Recipe 36

<u>Tofu, Avocado & Spinach Salad</u>

   3 tablespoons soy sauce
   4 cloves garlic, minced
   4 teaspoons Sriracha
   4 teaspoons sesame oil, divided
   1 block firm tofu, cut into 1-inch squares
   4 ounces baby spinach
   1 medium avocado, cut into small pieces
   1 medium cucumber, cut into small pieces

1) Marinate: In a large shallow bowl, whisk together soy sauce, garlic and Sriracha . Gently toss tofu in marinade. Arrange tofu in a single layer. Cover and refrigerate for at least 1 hour. Remove tofu and set aside marinade mixture.
2) Meanwhile add spinach, avocado and cucumber to 4 plates. Set aside.
3) After marinating tofu, heat 2 teaspoons of sesame oil in a skillet over medium-high heat. Add tofu and cook until tofu is golden brown on all sides.
4) Add tofu to plates with vegetables and drizzle with remainder of marinade mixture and remainder of sesame oil.

<u>Serves 4</u>. About 170 Calories per serving.

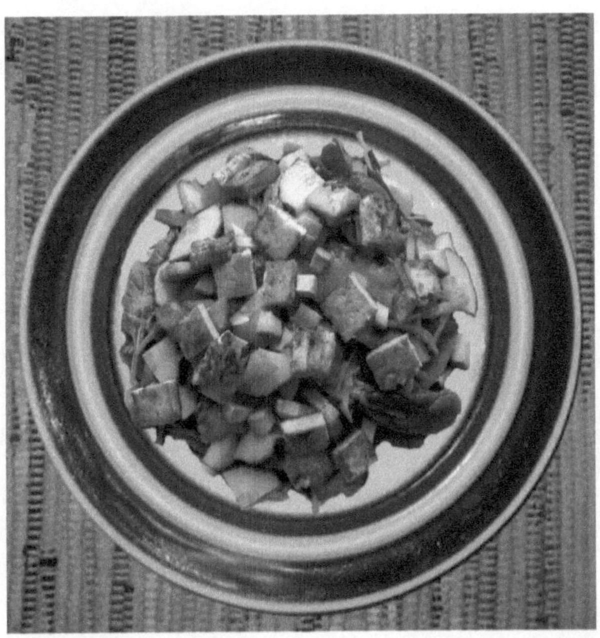

Suggest this dish be served with ½ cup brown rice. This adds 100 Calories per serving. But makes this a complete low-calorie meal.

43

Recipe 37

Tofu Steak & Veggie Stir Fry

15 ounces of extra-firm tofu
2   tablespoons peanut oil
1   teaspoon garlic, minced (1 to 2 cloves)
½   cup pecans, coarsely chopped
2   tablespoons brown sugar
3   tablespoons reduced-sodium soy sauce
¼   teaspoon crushed red pepper flakes (optional)
1   head broccoli, cut into florets
½   red bell pepper, cut into thin 1-inch long strips
½   red onion, thinly sliced

1) Press and drain tofu. Cut tofu into 3 crosswise slices, and cut each slice into 3 or 4 long strips.

2) In a large skillet, heat peanut oil over medium-high heat. Add tofu strips and cook without stirring for about 3 minutes, until they have browned on the bottom. Flip tofu and add garlic and pecans, stirring for a minute until the garlic becomes fragrant. Add sugar, 1½ tablespoons soy sauce, and red pepper flakes (if used) and stir until sugar blends with remainder of ingredients. Remove tofu and nuts to a plate, allowing some of the sauce to remain in pan.

3) Add broccoli, red pepper strips, onions, and remaining soy sauce and cook for 3 to 4 minutes, until tender. Add the tofu and other ingredients back into skillet to heat them through, and serve immediately.

Serves 4. About 310 Calories per serving.

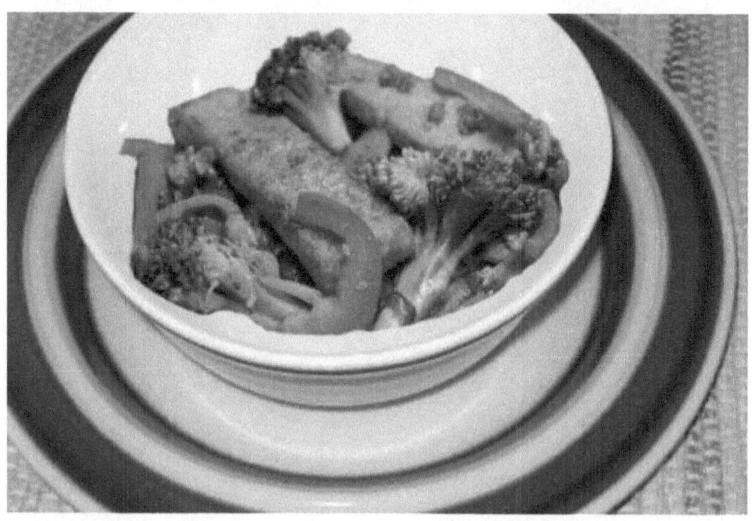

White Beans & Kale Vegan Soup

1 large yellow onion, chopped
2 teaspoons olive oil
3 garlic cloves, finely minced
64 ounces of vegetable stock
2 pounds Yukon gold potatoes, chopped
2 15-ounce cans cannellini beans
2 tablespoons fresh rosemary, finely chopped
3 cups kale, stems removed & torn into 2" pieces

1) Heat a large pot over medium heat with 2 teaspoons olive oil. Sauté onions for 5-7 minutes until translucent. Add in 1.5 tablespoons minced garlic and cook until fragrant, 1 minute.
2) Pour in vegetable stock, potatoes, cannellini beans and rosemary. Bring to a low boil, reduce heat to low and simmer uncovered for 30 minutes.
3) Add the kale to the soup and cook 5 more minutes. Remove from heat, salt & pepper to taste, then allow to rest for 5 minutes.

Serves 6. About 410 Calories per serving.

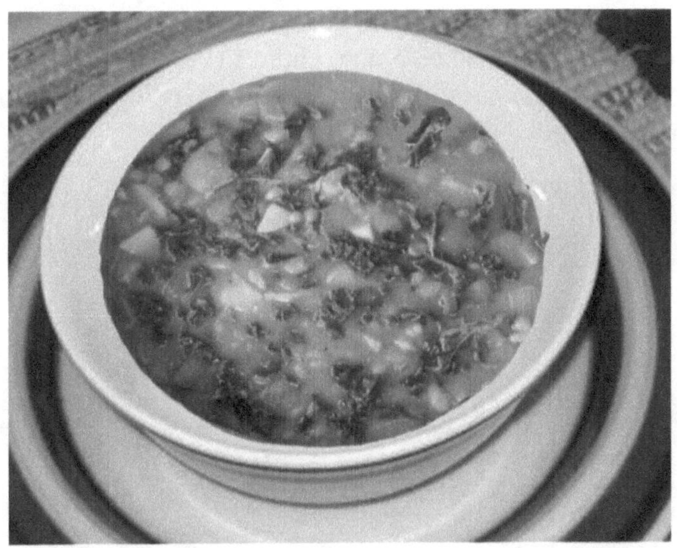

Recipe 39

<u>Low-Cal New England Clam Chowder</u>

4 cups cauliflower florets
2 cups low-fat milk
1 tablespoon olive oil
2 leeks, thinly sliced
2 celery stalks, chopped
1 cup radicchio, shredded
3 cups clam juice
1½ teaspoon dried thyme
1 bay leaf
1 cup canned chopped clams
3 medium potatoes, peeled, boiled, cut into chunks
1 tablespoon fresh parsley, chopped

1) Bring large pot of water to a boil; add cauliflower florets and cook until cauliflower is tender, about 10 to15 minutes; drain well. Place in blender with milk and puree until smooth.
2) Heat olive oil in soup pot. Add leeks and celery stalk to soup pot. Sauté until leeks are softened; add clam juice, thyme and bay leaf. Season to taste with salt and pepper. Bring to a boil. Whisk in pureed cauliflower and milk mixture. Add clams and cooked potato chunks (if using) cook until clams are just cooked through, about 5 minutes. Stir in parsley just before serving.
3) Ladle soup into bowls and garnish with radicchio.

<u>Serves 6</u>. About 180 Calories per serving.

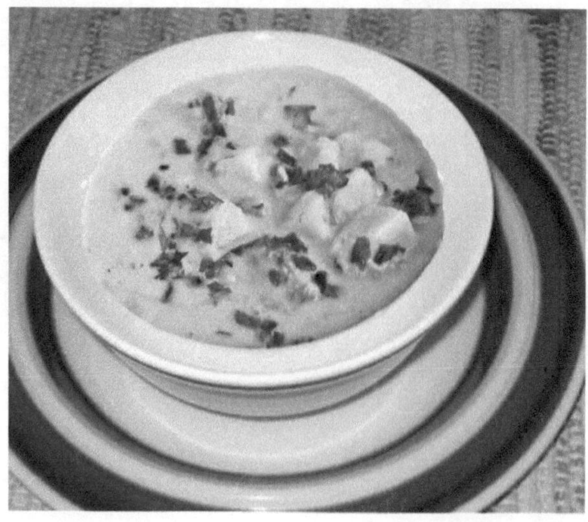

Noodle Soup with Bok Choy & Egg

 4   cups vegetable broth
 2   whole star anise
 1   stick whole cinnamon
 2   large eggs
 ½ 7.8-ounce package udon noodles
 4   large bok choy leaves, sliced into ribbons
 2   scallions, thinly sliced 5
 3   tablespoons soy sauce

1) In a medium saucepan bring vegetable broth to a simmer. Add star anise and cinnamon stick and simmer for 5 to 10 minutes to infuse broth with spices. When finished, use a slotted spoon to remove spices.

2) Crack eggs into separate measuring cups and slip them into simmering broth, one at a time. Cook for 2 minutes, then add noodles and bok choy. Stir very gently to submerge the noodles and bok choy, but do not break the eggs. Simmer for another 2 minutes, until the whites of the eggs are completely set but the yolks are still loose.

3) Turn off heat and gently stir in soy sauce and spring onions. Divide soup between four bowls and serve immediately.

Serves 2. About 360 Calories per serving.

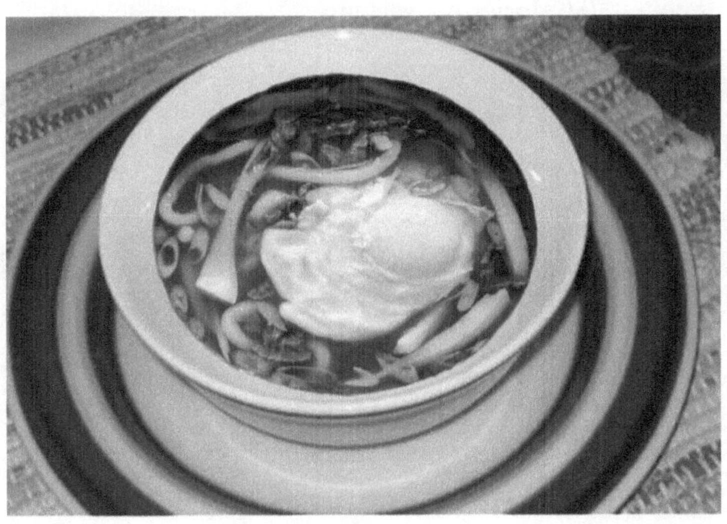

Recipe 41

Asian Noodles & Shrimp Stir Fry

    1   7.8-ounce package of udon noodles
    3   tablespoons of soy sauce
    ¼   cup of oyster sauce
    1   clove garlic, chopped
    1   teaspoon ginger, grated
    ¼   cup vegetable broth
    1   teaspoon sugar
    2   tablespoons vegetable oil
    4   cups mixed vegetables*
    24 medium shrimp

1) Wash vegetables and cut into pieces. Set aside.
2) Cook noodles per package directions. Set aside.
3) Combine soy sauce, oyster sauce, vegetable broth and sugar in a small bowl. Set aside.
4) In large skillet or wok heat 1 tablespoon of oil over low heat. Add noodles and sauce mixture. Toss and cook about 5 minutes.
5) Add another tablespoon of oil and then the ginger and garlic. Stir and then cook shrimp. Once shrimp are cooked, add vegetables and stir for about 5 to 7 minutes.

Serves 4. About 430 Calories per serving.

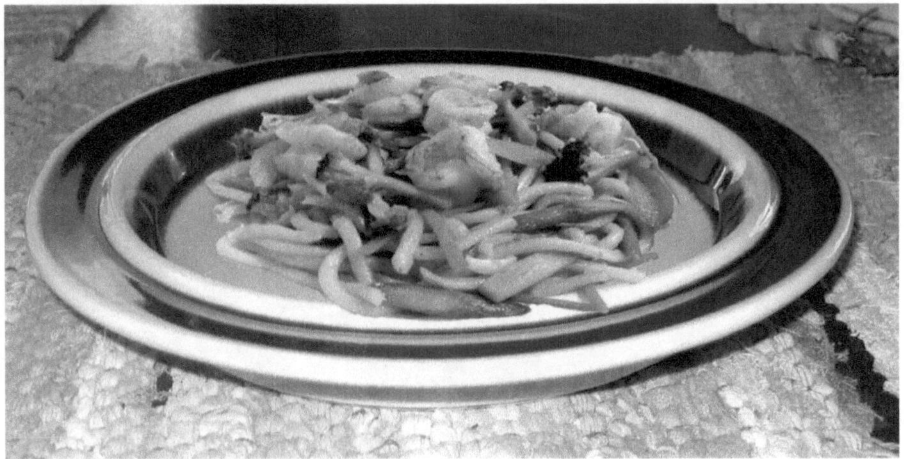

* Vegetable mix: broccoli, carrots and asparagus cut as shown.

Recipe 42

<u>Scallop & Noodle Stir Fry</u>

  1 tablespoon vegetable oil
  2 tablespoons minced ginger
  2 tablespoons minced garlic
  1 pound sea scallops, halved
  8 ounces snow peas
½ cup lower sodium vegetable broth
  3 tablespoons soy sauce
  2 tablespoons green onion, chopped
  6 ounces thin egg noodles

1) Cook noodles according to package directions.
2) Meanwhile, in a large non-stick skillet (or wok), heat vegetable oil over medium-high heat. Add garlic and ginger and cook, stirring, until fragrant, about 30 seconds.
3) Add scallops and stir to coat with garlic mixture and cook about 1 minute. Mix in snow peas and cook another minute. Stir in vegetable broth and soy sauce and cook until just simmering.
4) Sprinkle with green onions, mix with noodles and serve.

<u>Serves 4</u>. About 325 Calories per serving.

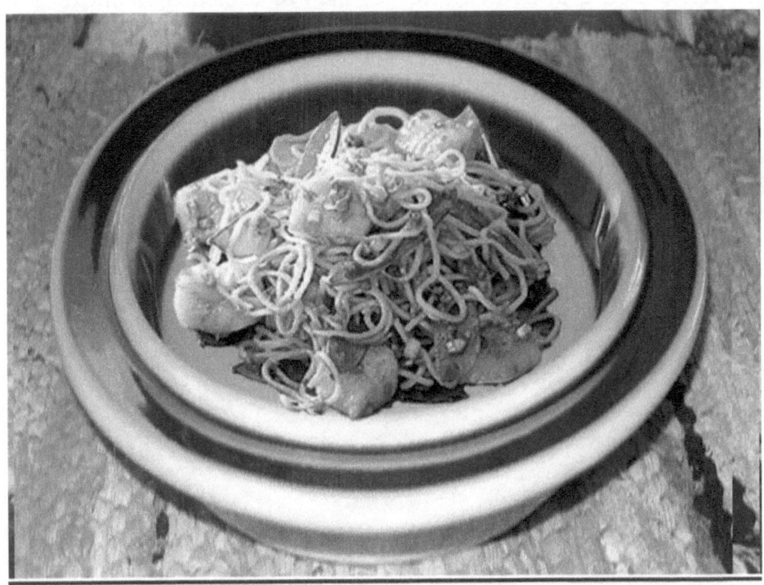

Recipe 43

<u>Swordfish with Veggies</u>

   1¼ pounds swordfish
   1 bottle citrus-herb marinade
   12 broccoli florets
   1 bunch of asparagus
   2 ripe medium-size tomatoes
   2 tablespoons Lo-Cal (light) salad dressing

Place evenly cut broccoli and asparagus spears in a microwave-safe pan, add a little water to bottom of the pan and top with microwave-safe plastic wrap. (Be sure to pull back one corner of the plastic topper so some steam can escape.) Check veggies periodically and take them out of the microwave when they reach desired softness.

Immerse swordfish in marinade. Grill on hot fire for about 5 minutes on one side and 3 minutes on the other, or until done as desired

For each serving, plate about ¼ of swordfish and a portion of the steamed broccoli and asparagus. Add one-half of a tomato cut into pieces. Drizzle about 2 tablespoons of low-calorie salad dressing that contains no more than 25 Calories per tablespoon.

<u>Serves 4</u>: One serving of swordfish, veggies & dressing is about 310 Calories.

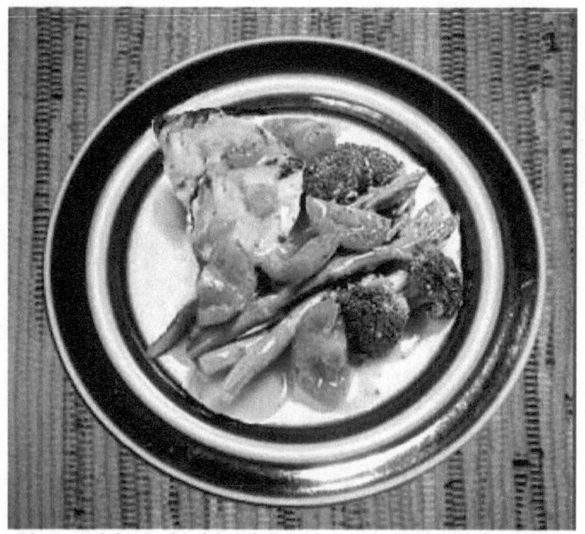

Shown drizzled with Light Thousand Island dressing.

Tilapia Piccata

    4 tilapia filets (about 6 ounces each)
    2 teaspoons olive oil
    1 teaspoon minced garlic
    ¼ cup shallots, diced
    ¾ pound fresh green beans, washed and snipped
    1 teaspoon lemon juice
    ¼ cup capers, rinsed
    2 fresh lemons, cut into small wedges

In a skillet, heat olive oil and minced garlic over medium heat. Sauté tilapia and shallots for two to three minutes, tossing often, until tilapia is partially cooked. Add green beans and one teaspoon of lemon juice and sauté for an additional two to three minutes, or until tilapia is completely cooked and green beans are al dente. Add capers; and cover tilapia. Let sit for one more minute to warm capers. Serve immediately with wedges of lemon.

<u>**Serves 4**</u>. 330 calories per serving

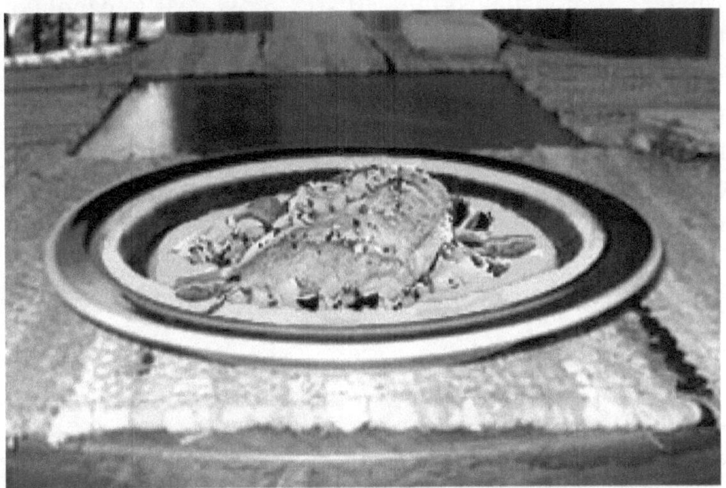

Note: We suggest this dish be accompanied by ½ cup cooked brown rice and a large tossed salad with 1½ tablespoons of low-cal dressing. This adds about 170 Calories. Then the total for the plate is 500 Calories.

Recipe 45

<u>Hoisin Shrimp Stir Fry</u>

Hoisin sauce is a thick, pungent sauce often used in Chinese cooking as a glaze or an addition to a stir fry.

    1 tablespoon cornstarch
    ⅓ cup reduced-sodium vegetable broth
    4½ teaspoons reduced-sodium soy sauce
    4½ teaspoons hoisin sauce
    1 teaspoon sesame oil
    1 tablespoon canola oil
    3 ounces snow peas, halved
    4 green onions, chopped
    3 garlic cloves, minced
    1 teaspoon minced fresh gingerroot
    1 pound uncooked medium shrimp, peeled and deveined

1) In a small bowl, combine cornstarch and broth until smooth. Stir in soy sauce, hoisin sauce and sesame oil; set aside.

2) In a large wok or nonstick skillet, stir-fry snow peas in canola oil until crisp-tender. Add onions, garlic and ginger; stir-fry for 3-4 minutes or until vegetables are tender. Add shrimp; stir-fry 4-5 minutes longer or until shrimp turn pink.

3) Stir cornstarch mixture and add to the pan. Bring to a boil; cook and stir for 2 minutes or until thickened.

<u>**Serves 4**</u>. 200 calories per serving

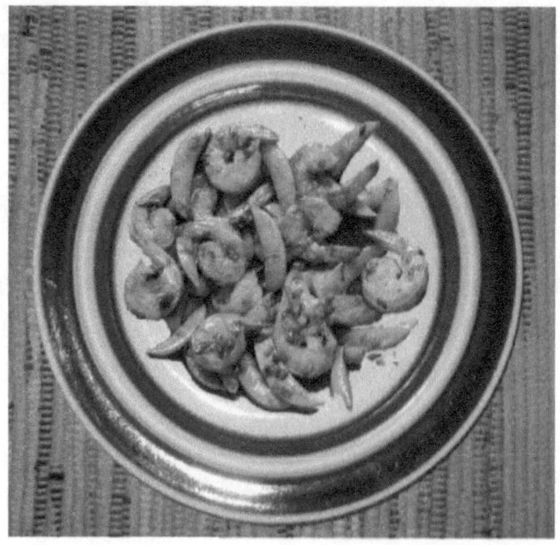

Note: We suggest this dish served over ½ cup cooked brown rice. Then the total for the plate is 300 Calories.

52

Recipe 46

<u>Healthy Tuna Salad</u>

2	7-oz cans solid white albacore tuna 420
2	beefsteak tomatoes, cut into pieces 70
1	celery heart, chopped 30
¼	pound roasted red peppers, from jar, chopped 100
1	small red onion, peeled, halved 20
10	black olives, halved 100
1	small bunch basil, leaves only
1½	tablespoons red wine vinegar 20
3	tablespoons extra-virgin olive oil 330
¼	pound croutons 400

Break up tuna and mix with croutons, tomatoes, celery, roasted peppers, red onion, olives and basil in large bowl and season with salt and black pepper. Drizzle with 3 tablespoons extra-virgin olive oil and balsamic vinegar and toss.

<u>Serves 4.</u> 370 Calories per serving

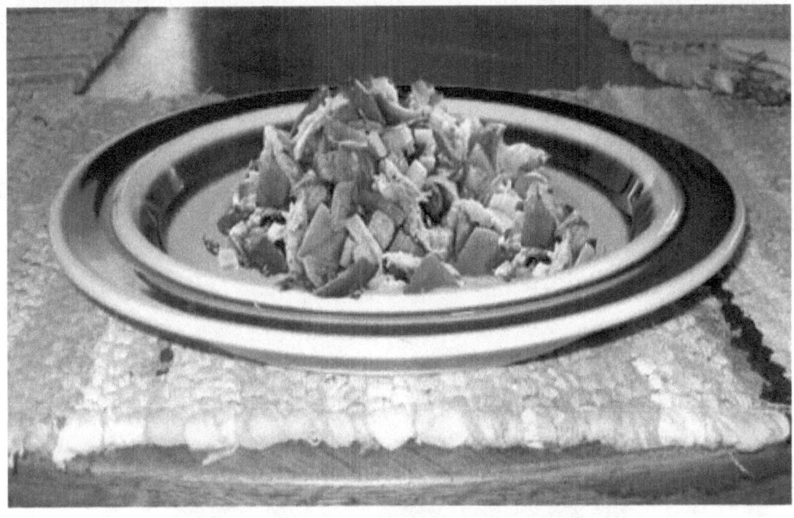

Recipe 47

Salmon Patties

2 tablespoons mayonnaise
1 tablespoon lemon juice
1½ teaspoons Dijon mustard
¼ cup finely chopped green onions
2 tablespoons minced red bell pepper
½ teaspoon garlic powder
¼ teaspoon salt
⅛ teaspoon ground red pepper
2 (6-ounce) packages skinless, boneless pink salmon
1 large egg, lightly beaten
1 cup panko breadcrumbs
1 tablespoon canola oil
1 tablespoon chopped fresh parsley
1 teaspoon finely chopped capers
½ teaspoon minced garlic

1. Combine mayonnaise, lemon juice, mustard and next 7 ingredients (through egg), stirring well. Add breadcrumbs and toss. Shape mixture into 8 (3-inch diameter) patties.
2. Heat oil in a large skillet over medium heat. Add patties; cook 5 minutes on each side or until browned.
3. Place 2 patties on bed of mixed salad greens. Drizzle with 1 tablespoon low-calorie dressing.

Serves 4. About 350 Calories per serving (includes salad and dressing*).

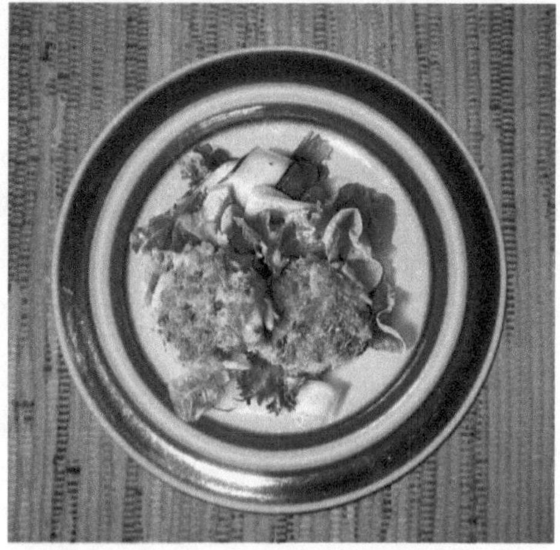

* Use a low-calorie dressing that contains no more than 25 Calories per tablespoon.

Recipe 48

<u>Baked Herb-Crusted Cod</u>

    4 cod fish fillets (4 to 5 ounces each)
    2 tablespoons all-purpose flour
    2 tablespoons cornmeal
    2 tablespoons minced fresh herbs
    2 teaspoons lemon juice

Sprinkle cod with lemon juice. Mix flour, cornmeal and herbs and dust the cod with the cornmeal-herb mixture. Bake in oven at 375 °F for 10 minutes. Add salt and black pepper to taste.

<u>Serves 4</u>. One serving is about 230 Calories (for cod only).

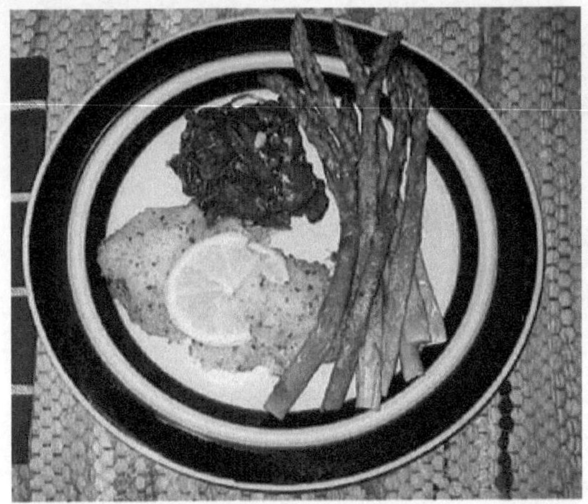

Note: The spinach cooked with garlic and drizzled with olive oil and the steamed asparagus spears add about 125 Calories. Then the total for the plate, as shown, is 355 Calories.

Baked Salmon with Salsa

This is a simple, straight-forward recipe. The advantage of a simple recipe is there are no hidden calories.

    4   5 oz salmon fillets
    6   tablespoons bottled salsa

Brown salmon fillets in non-stick pan and then place them in a baking dish. Cook fillets in an oven preheated to 350 ºF for about 10 minutes. Plate the salmon. Stir bottled tomato-pepper salsa and spoon it over the salmon. **Serves 4**. One salmon fillet is about 215 Calories.

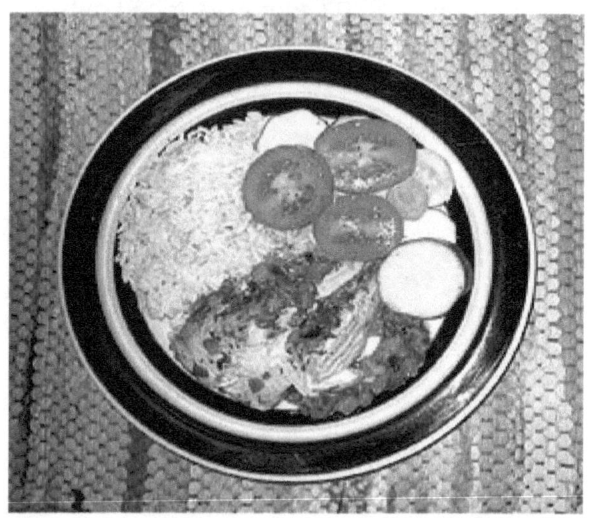

Note: The baked summer squash, brown rice and sliced tomato add about 160 Calories. Then the total for the plate, as shown, is about 375 Calories.

Recipe 50

Red Snapper with Yogurt Sauce

    4   4-ounce red snapper fillets (salmon fillets okay)
    ½ cup white wine
    ½ cup non-fat plain yogurt mixed with ¼ cup mustard
    ½ pound green beans
    ¾ pint cherry tomatoes (about 20), halved
    4 teaspoons olive oil
    ¾ cup wild rice, brown rice and wheat berry mix.

Brown fillets in non-stick pan. Place fillets skin side down in baking dish coated with non-stick spray. Add white wine and cook in oven preheated to 350 ºF for about 15 minutes . Spoon pan juices over fillets. Salt and pepper to taste.

Place green beans in skillet. Add ¼-inch of water and cook over medium heat until water boils off. Add cherry tomatoes and olive oil. Stir well and sauté for a few minutes. (If desired, season with fresh rosemary and oregano.) Salt and pepper to taste.

Prepare rice mix per package directions

Plate red snapper fillet and spoon over yogurt-mustard sauce. Add green beans and tomato mix and the wild rice mix. Serve hot.

Serves 4. One plate consisting of one snapper fillet (215 Calories) with green beans and tomato mix (75 Calories) and wild rice (160 Calories) totals 450 Calories.

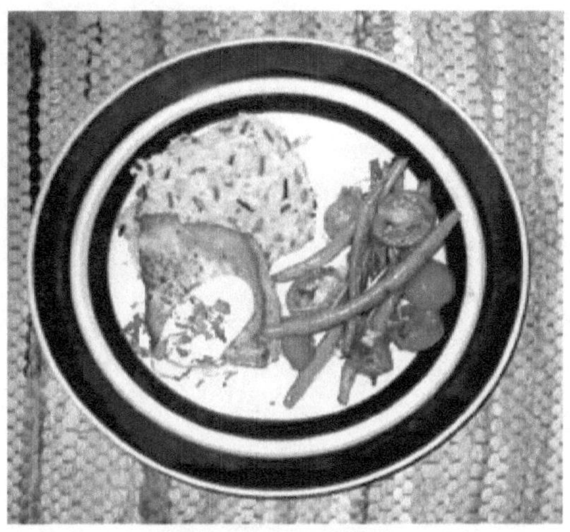

Recipe 51

<u>Grilled Swordfish</u>

    1¼ pounds swordfish
    1 bottle citrus-herb marinade
    ¾ pint cherry tomatoes (about 20), halved
    4 medium potatoes
    2 cups fresh spinach
    1 teaspoon rosemary & juice of ¼ lemon
    2 teaspoon extra-virgin olive oil, divided

Steam spinach with garlic and drizzle with about 1 teaspoon extra-virgin olive oil.

Cut potatoes in medium-size pieces and sprinkle with lemon juice, add rosemary, salt and black pepper. Place potatoes on grill for about 10 minutes, turning occasionally.

Toss cherry tomatoes in remaining extra-virgin olive oil. Add fresh oregano, salt and black pepper. Place on heavy-duty aluminum foil, seal and grill for about 3 minutes.

<u>Lemon-Herb Marinade</u>: 1 lemon - juiced, 1 Tbsp olive oil, 2 garlic cloves minced, 1 tsp fresh thyme chopped, 1 tsp fresh oregano chopped & 1 tsp minced green onion

Immerse swordfish in marinade. Grill on hot fire for about 5 minutes on one side and 3 minutes on the other, or until done as desired

<u>**Serves 4**</u>. One plate of grilled swordfish (250 Calories) with potatoes (100 Calories), cherry tomatoes (45 Calories) and steamed spinach (50 Calories) totals 445 Calories.

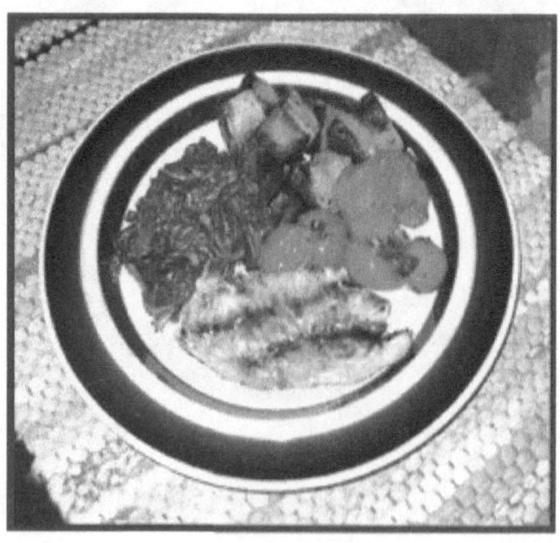

58

Recipe 52

<u>Shrimp & Spinach Salad</u>

- 2 pounds shrimp in shell
- ½ pound small green beans, trimmed
- ½ pound baby spinach leaves
- 2 tablespoon lemon juice
- ¼ cup extra-virgin olive oil
- 2 teaspoon minced fresh dill
- 1 tablespoon minced green onion

To make vinaigrette, combine lemon juice, olive oil, dill, salt and black pepper to taste and whisk until blended. Stir in minced onion and set aside. Steam green beans and set aside.

Peel, de-vein and butterfly shrimp. Place shrimp in a bowl and add water to cover. Add 1 teaspoon of salt, and let stand for 10 minutes. Drain, rinse, drain again, and dry. Arrange shrimp in broiling pan without a rack. Brush shrimp with a little of the vinaigrette and place under preheated broiler, about 3 inches from heat. Broil about 3 to 4 minutes, turning shrimp once, or until both sides turn pink.

Remove shrimp from broiler and add remaining vinaigrette and green beans to the broiling pan. Stir to coat shrimp and beans with vinaigrette. Pour warm vinaigrette over spinach and toss quickly. Plate the spinach and arrange shrimp and green beans on top.

<u>Serves 4</u>. 310 Calories per serving.

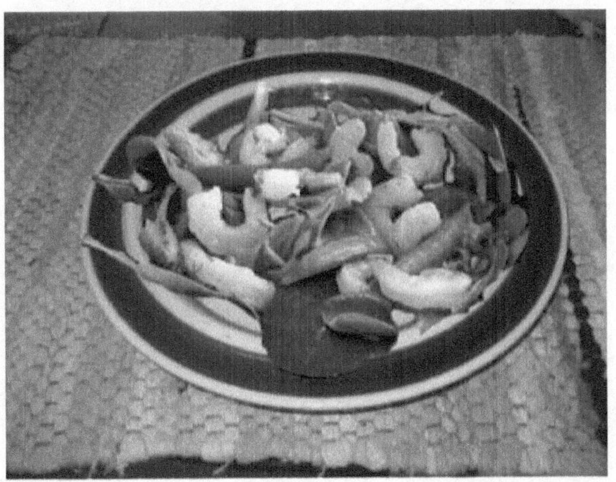

Recipe 53

<u>Tina's Grilled Scallops & Polenta</u>

    1 pound sea scallops
    ¾ cup polenta
    ¾ cup skim milk
    1 medium portobello mushroom
    ½ pound green beans
    ¼ cup chopped red onion
    16 asparagus spears
    1 teaspoon extra-virgin olive oil

Bring 1½ cups of water and skim milk to rapid boil. Add salt to taste and slowly add polenta while stirring. Reduce heat. Continue stirring until desired consistency is reached. Pour polenta into lightly greased pan. After polenta has cooled cover and refrigerate. Cut chilled polenta into 4 pieces. Grill on medium-hot fire – about two minutes on each side.

Brush portobello mushroom and asparagus spears with olive oil and place on grill for about 3 minutes on each side.

Grill scallops on medium-hot fire. Turn after two minutes or when first side turns opaque. Grill until second side turns opaque – about another 2 minutes. Don't overcook but test a scallop by cutting to make sure it's cooked through. Salt and pepper to taste.

<u>Serves 4.</u> The food on the plate pictured below totals about 380 Calories.

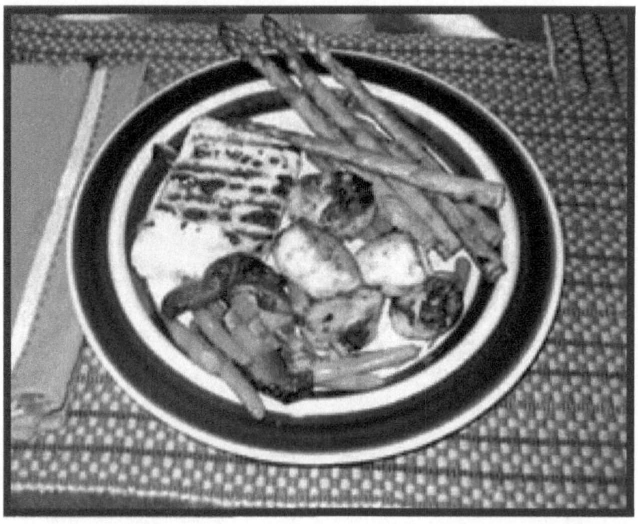

Recipe 54

Baked Sea Bass

    4 4-ounce Chilean sea bass fillets
    ½ pound green beans
    ¾ pint cherry tomatoes (about 20)
    ¾ cup brown rice (prepare per package directions)

Sea Bass: Dust filets with all-purpose flour. Dip in egg wash and then Panko breadcrumbs. Place fillets in baking dish coated with non-stick spray. Bake about 15 minutes in oven preheated to 350 ºF.

Green Beans & Tomato: Place green beans in skillet. Add ¼-inch of water and cook over medium heat until water boils off. Add cherry tomatoes and olive oil. Stir well and sauté for a few minutes. Season with fresh rosemary and oregano.

Brown Rice-Pesto mix: Prepare brown rice per package directions. Add 4 teaspoons packaged "green" pesto*. Mix thoroughly.

Red Pepper Sauce: Blend one roasted red pepper (skinned), ½ cup non-fat plain yogurt, 1 tsp lemon juice, 1 Tbsp olive oil, 1 Tbsp chili sauce, and a dash of Worcestershire sauce.

Serves 4. One plate consisting of one sea bass fillet with spooned over red pepper sauce (150 Calories), green beans & tomato mix (75 Calories), brown rice-pesto mix (120 Calories) and half ear of corn (50 Calories) – totals about 395 Calories.

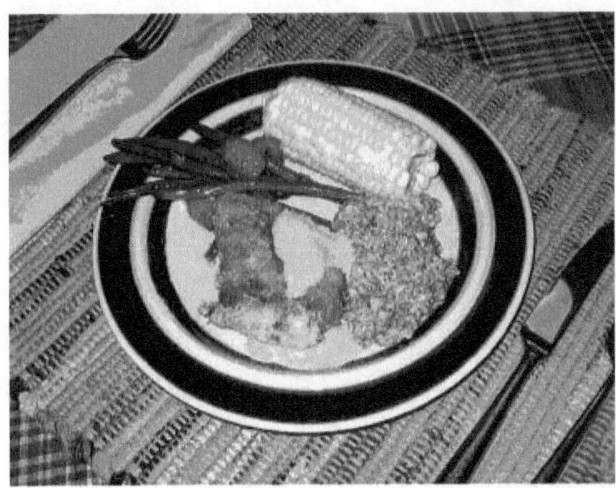

Recipe 55

<u>Grilled Tilapia</u>

Tilapia is a mild, white fish that inhabits fresh water. This fish has very low levels of mercury because it's fast-growing, short-lived, and mostly eats a vegetarian diet. According to the Monterey Bay Aquarium, choose tilapia farmed in the U.S., in environmentally friendly systems. "Avoid" farmed tilapia from China and Taiwan, where pollution and weak management are a problem.

   4 Tilapia filets (about 6 ounces each)

<u>Marinade</u>: ¾ cup olive oil, ½ lemon, juiced, 1 tablespoons oregano, ½ teaspoon black pepper, ¼ cup red wine vinegar, ½ cup finely chopped parsley, 2 cloves garlic, minced.

Combine all ingredients (except filets) in a large re-sealable plastic bag and shake well. Then place fish filets in the marinade for 30 minutes. Remove fillets from marinade and cook on hot grill for approximately 2 to 3 minutes per side.

<u>Serves 4.</u> About 300 Calories per serving (fish only)

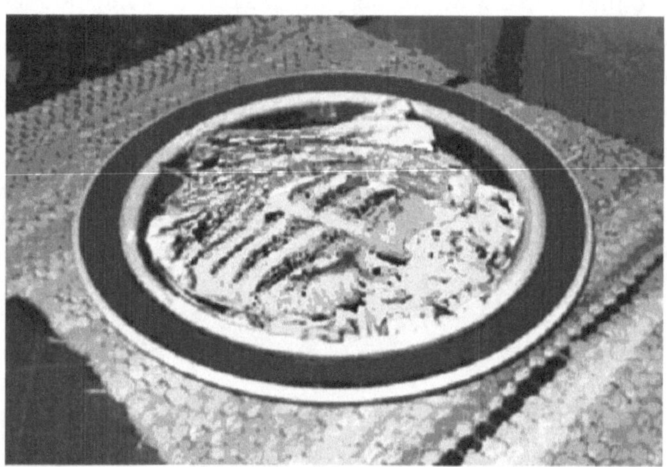

Photo shows two fish filets. Actual serving size is <u>one filet</u>.

Note: Six asparagus spears and ½ up cooked wild rice adds about 125 Calories. Then the total for the plate, with one fish fillet, is 425 Calories.

__Baked Haddock__

  4 4-oz haddock fillets (or salmon fillets)
  ½ cup white wine
  ½ cup white wine
  ½ cup non-fat yogurt mixed with ¼ cup pureed roasted red pepper
  ½ pound green beans
  ¾ pint cherry tomatoes (about 20)
  1 tablespoon olive oil
  ¾ cup quinoa, prepared per package directions

Lightly dust fillets with flour. Dip in beaten egg white and then in Panko bread crumbs. Brown fillets in non-stick pan. Place fillets skin side down in baking dish coated with non-stick spray. Add white wine and cook in oven preheated to 350 ºF for about 15 minutes. Spoon pan juices over fillets. Salt and pepper to taste.

Place green beans in skillet. Add ¼-inch of water and cook over medium heat until water boils off. Add cherry tomatoes and olive oil. Stir well and sauté for a few minutes. Season with fresh rosemary and oregano. Salt and pepper to taste.

Plate haddock fillet and spoon over yogurt-red pepper sauce. Garnish with fresh parsley. Add green beans & tomato mix and the quinoa. Serve hot.

__Serves 4__. One plate consisting of one haddock fillet (215 Calories) with green beans & tomato mix (65 Calories) and quinoa (120 Calories) totals 400 Calories.

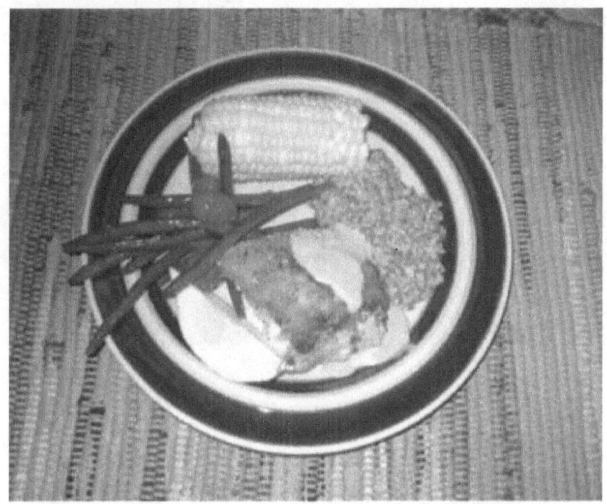

Corn-on-the-cob is only for the 1,800 Calorie diet.

Poached Cod in Tomato Broth

  2 cups dry white wine
  1 cup clam juice
  2 cans (14.5-ounce) diced tomatoes, drained
  1 small onion, diced
  1 garlic clove, minced
  ½ tsp dried parsley, or sprigs of fresh parsley
  1 bay leaf
12 black olives, pitted and halved
  4 cod fish fillets (about 6 ounces each)
Note that sole, flounder, halibut or haddock may be substituted for cod.

Use a pan large enough to hold the fish in a single layer. Place all the ingredients except the fish in the pan. Over high heat, bring poaching liquid to a boil (pan uncovered). Reduce heat and simmer the liquid another 6 minutes.

Carefully place the fish filets in the liquid. Cover the pan and reduce heat until liquid is just simmering. Poach until fish are completely opaque and tender – about 8 minutes. Plate fish and ladle broth over fish.

Serves 4. 275 Calories per serving.

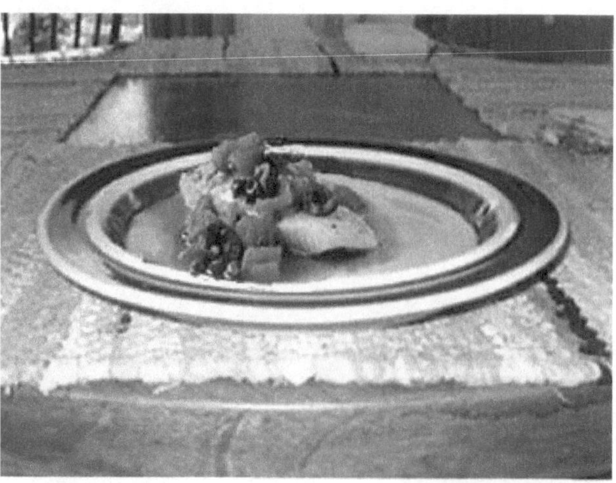

Recipe 58

<u>Barbequed Shrimp & Corn</u>

   1½ pounds large shrimp, peeled and de-veined
   3 Tbsp of bottled barbeque sauce
   4 medium ears of corn

Pour barbeque sauce into shallow bowl. Toss shrimp in barbeque sauce to coat. Place shrimp on medium-hot grill. Turn shrimp after about two minutes or when shrimp turn pink. Grill until second side turns pink – approximately another 2 minutes. Don't overcook but test a shrimp by cutting to make sure it is cooked through. Salt and pepper to taste. Serve hot or at room temperature.

<u>**Serves 4**</u>. About 160 Calories per serving (shrimp only).

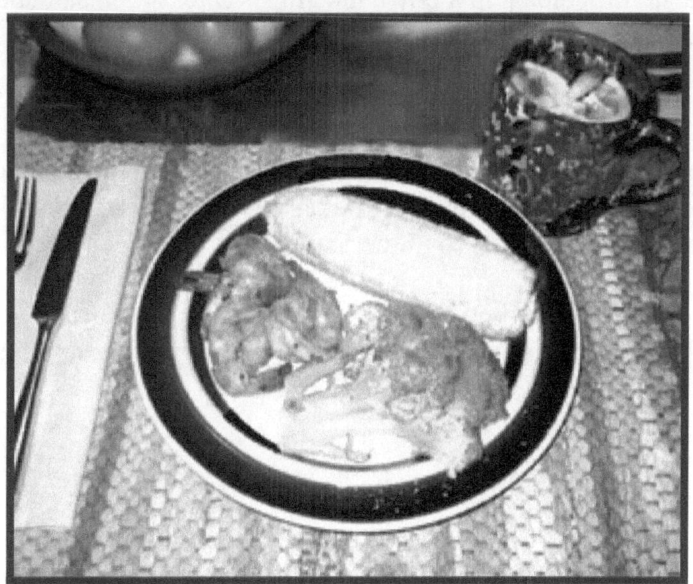

Note: The corn on the cob and one cup of steamed broccoli add about 140 Calories. Then the total for the plate, as shown, is 300 Calories.

<h1 style="text-align: center;">Recipe 59</h1>

Pan-Fried Sole

    4   sole fillets (6-ounces each), skinned
    1   tablespoon olive oil

Salsa Ingredients:

    1 pint cherry tomatoes, quartered
    ¾ cup cucumber, finely chopped
    ⅓ cup yellow bell pepper, finely chopped
    3 tablespoons fresh basil, chopped
    2 tablespoons capers
    1½ tablespoons shallots, finely chopped
    1 tablespoon balsamic vinegar
    2 teaspoons lemon rind, grated

Combine salsa ingredients in a bowl and stir in ½ teaspoon salt and ⅛ teaspoon black pepper. Mix thoroughly.

Heat olive oil in a large nonstick skillet over medium-high heat. Season sole fillets with
½ teaspoon salt and ⅛ teaspoon black pepper. Add fish to pan; cook about 1½ minutes on each side or until fish flakes easily when tested with a fork. Spoon salsa over fish and serve immediately.

Serves 4. 325 Calories per serving

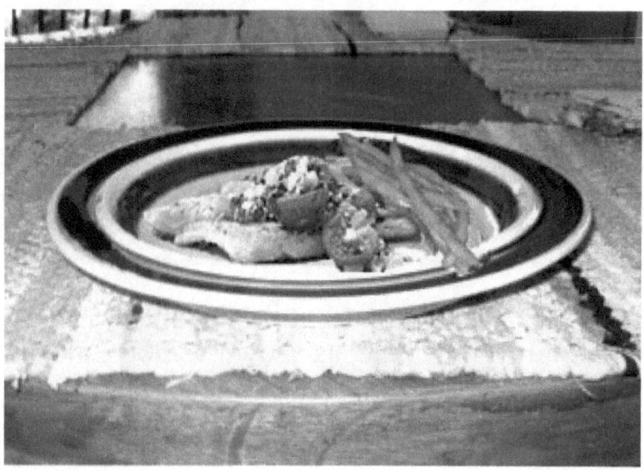

Recipe 60

<u>Salmon with Mango Salsa</u>

    4 salmon fillets (about 5 ounces each)
    1½ pounds baby new potatoes, halved
    1 mango, ripe
    3 green onions, finely chopped
    3 tablespoons chopped fresh cilantro
    2 tablespoons lemon juice
    2 teaspoons extra-virgin olive oil
    4 cups watercress

Remove any tiny bones from salmon. Press crushed peppercorns into flesh side of salmon. Set aside. Place halved potatoes into saucepan. Cover with water and bring to a boil. Reduce the heat and simmer until tender, about 10-12 minutes and drain.

Prepare salsa: Peel and seed the mango. Dice the mango flesh and put into a large bowl. Mix in green onions, cilantro, lemon juice, olive oil, and an optional dash of Tabasco.

Heat a grill pan coated with nonstick cooking spray over medium-high heat. Place salmon fillets in pan, skin-side down. Cook for 4 minutes. Turn fish over and cook until done, about another 4 minutes. Arrange watercress and new potatoes on serving plates. Place salmon on top and spoon over mango salsa.

<u>Serves 4</u>. 460 Calories per serving

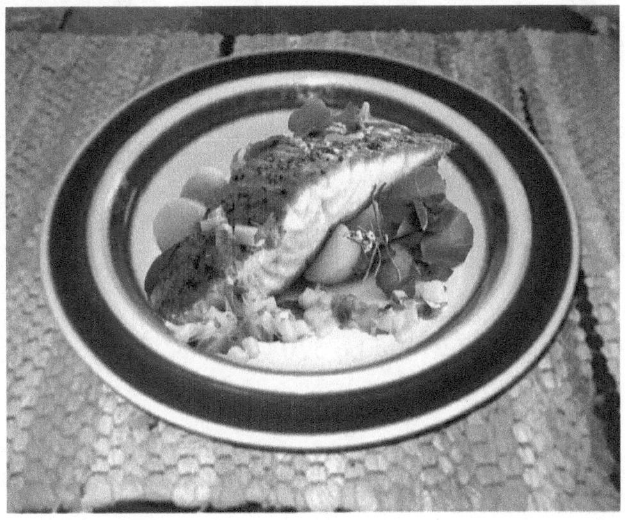

Recipe 61

<u>Shrimp over Spaghetti</u>

½ lb spaghetti
1 lb shrimp, peeled and de-veined
6 ounces dry white wine
3 tablespoons olive oil
3 cloves garlic, sliced thin
¼ cup chopped basil leaves

Cook spaghetti according to package directions. Save ½ cup of the pasta cooking water.

In a large skillet over medium heat, cook olive oil and garlic, stirring until garlic turns golden, and then discard garlic. Add shrimp and increase heat to medium-high and stir in chopped basil leaves, white wine and ½ cup cooking water. Cook another 2 to 3 minutes or until shrimp are just firm. Spoon shrimp and sauce over spaghetti. Season with salt and black pepper. Garnish with parsley.

<u>Serves 4</u>. 450 Calories per serving

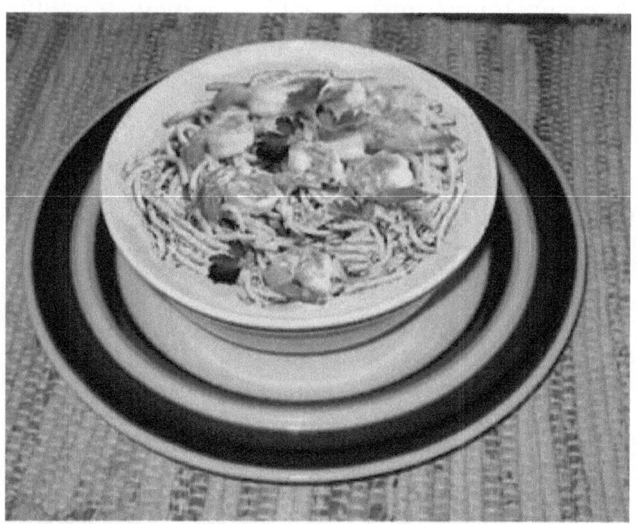

Note: Have a large tossed salad which adds about 70 Calories to the meal. Then the total for this meal would be 520 Calories.

Recipe 62

Baked Cod

    4 cod fish fillets (4 to 5 ounces each)
    2 tablespoons flour
    2 tablespoons cornmeal
    2 tablespoons minced fresh herbs
    2 teaspoons lemon juice

Sprinkle cod with lemon juice. Mix flour, cornmeal and herbs and dust the cod with the cornmeal-herb mixture. Bake in oven at 375 °F for 10 minutes. Add salt and black pepper to taste.

Serves 4. One serving is 230 Calories (cod only).

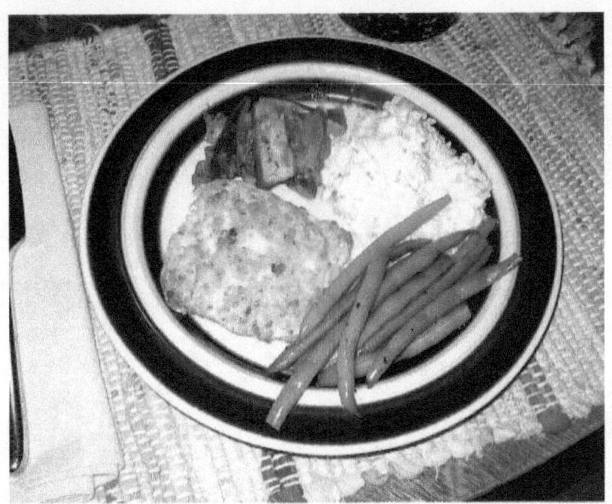

Note: The steamed green beans, steamed zucchini, tomatoes and onion mix, and ½ cup of cooked brown rice add about 170 Calories to the dish. Then the total for the meal shown is about 400 Calories.

Recipe 63

<u>Grilled Scallops</u>

We were invited by our good friends, Gary and Sue, for dinner. They prepared a simple, but nutritious low-calorie meal – which featured scallops. (Scallops are a very low calorie food – expensive but great when you're on a diet.) The photo below is our version of the main course they served that night.

    1½   pounds sea scallops
    3   medium tomatoes, sliced, divided
    4   ears of corn
    2   tablespoons olive oil, divided
    1   tablespoon balsamic vinegar, divided

Place scallops in a shallow bowl. Add olive oil and vinegar and toss to coat. Grill scallops on medium-hot fire. Turn after two minutes or when first side turns opaque. Grill until second side turns opaque – about another 2 minutes. Don't overcook but test a scallop by cutting to make sure it's cooked through. Salt and black pepper to taste.

<u>Serves 4</u>. The food pictured on the plate below totals about 360 Calories.

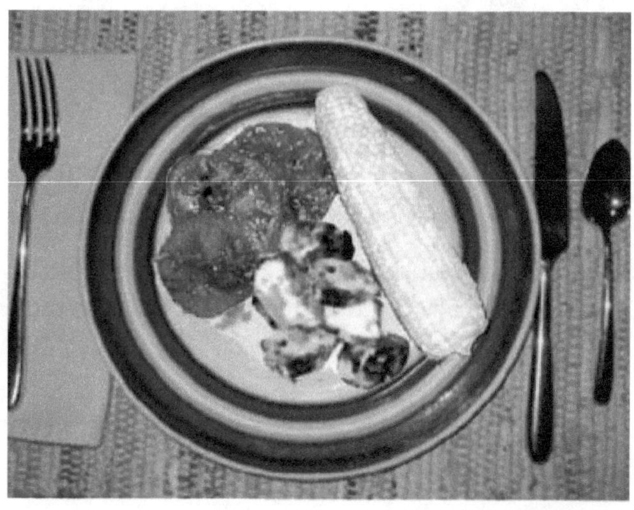

<u>Fish Stew</u>

1	pound shrimp, peeled and de-veined
¾	pound skinless flounder fillet, cut into strips
1	pound new baby potatoes, halved
2	peppers (red and yellow) sliced into strips
1	onion, halved and sliced
4	ounces white wine
2	cups lower sodium vegetable stock
2	cloves garlic, crushed
1	small bunch basil, shredded
1½	tablespoons olive oil

In a large pot, sauté garlic, onion and peppers in olive oil until they are completely softened. Stir in wine, vegetable stock and potatoes. Simmer until potatoes are tender.

Add the shrimp and flounder and cook for additional 4 minutes. Stir in basil and serve.

<u>**Serves 4**</u>. 300 Calories per serving

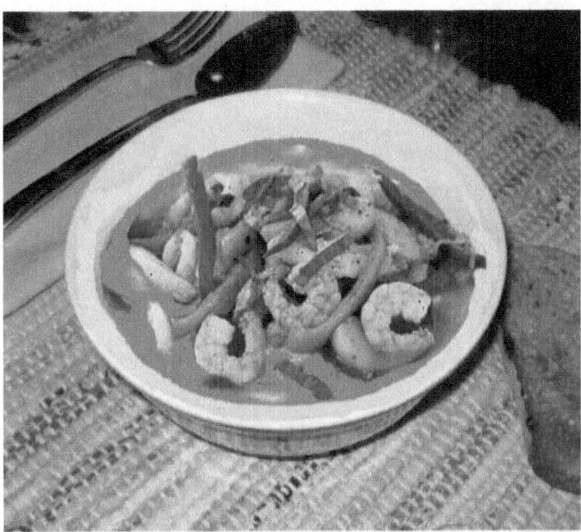

Note: Serve the fish stew with a large tossed salad (with 1½ tablespoons of low-calorie dressing). This adds about 70 Calories. Then the total for this meal is 370 Calories.

Recipe 65

<u>Trout with Lemon & Capers</u>

 4   trout fillets (4-oz each), skin attached
 3   tablespoons unsalted butter, divided
 2   tablespoons olive oil
 2   tablespoons lemon juice
 4   teaspoons chopped parsley
 1   teaspoon capers
 2   small lemons peeled and segmented

Score 2 crosswise slits (skin deep only) into each trout fillet using sharp knife. Turn the fillets over and season flesh with the salt and pepper.

Heat 1 tablespoon butter and the olive oil in a large nonstick skillet over medium-high heat. Place the fillets in the nonstick skillet, skin side up, and cook until golden brown, about 3 minutes. Turn and continue until cooked through and the skin begins to crisp around edges, about 2 more minutes. Transfer fillets to serving dish and keep warm.

Add the remaining 2 tablespoons butter to the hot skillet and cook until just brown. Stir in the lemon juice, parsley, capers, and lemon segments. Pour sauce over fillets and serve.

<u>Serves 4</u>. 340 Calories per serving (trout and sauce only)

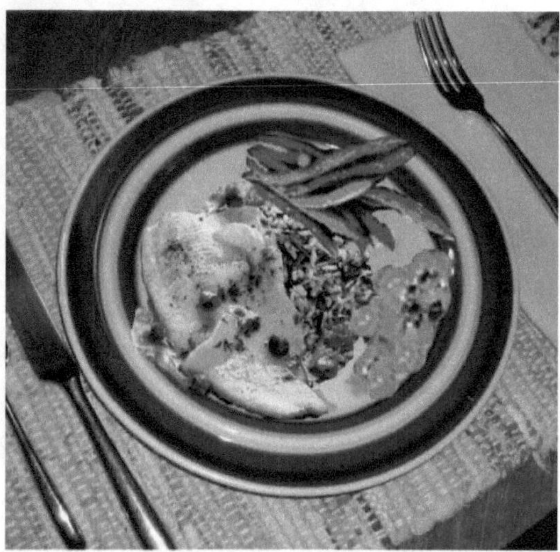

Note: The steamed green beans, sautéed cherry tomatoes, and ½ cup of cooked wild rice add about 190 Calories to the dish. Then the total for the meal shown is about 430 Calories.

<u>Tuna & Bean Salad</u>

    1   tuna steak, about 2 inches thick (14 ounces)
    2   tablespoons extra-virgin olive oil
    1   tablespoon lemon juice
    1   garlic clove, crushed
    1   tablespoon mustard
    1   15-ounce can cannellini beans, drained
    1   small red onion, thinly sliced
    2   red peppers, seeded and thinly sliced
    ½   cucumber, halved lengthwise and thinly sliced
    6   cups watercress

Heat a ridged grill pan coated with cooking spray over medium-high heat. Season tuna steak on both sides with coarsely ground black pepper. Cook the tuna 4 minutes on each side - the outside should be browned and the center light pink. Be careful not to overcook. Remove from the pan and set aside.

Mix together the oil, lemon juice, garlic, and mustard in a salad bowl. Season with salt and pepper to taste. Add the cannellini beans, onion, peppers, cucumber and watercress. Toss gently to mix. Cut tuna into ½-inch thick slices. Arrange on top of salad and serve with lemon wedges.

<u>Serves 4</u>. 355 Calories per serving

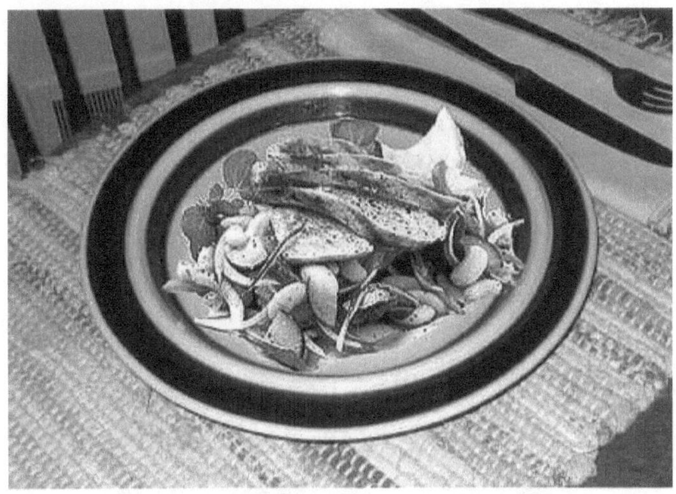

Recipe 67

<u>Crab Cakes</u>

    1   lb jumbo crab meat
    1½ Tbsp light mayonnaise
    1½ Tbsp chopped green bell pepper
    2   medium green onions, chopped
    1   large egg, beaten
    1   cup panko bread crumbs
    2   Tbsp canola oil
    ¼   tsp black pepper

Drain crab meat on layers of paper towels. Combine crab meat, bell pepper, mayonnaise, black pepper, onions and egg. Stir in ¼ cup panko bread crumbs. (Place remaining panko in shallow dish.)

Divide crab meat mixture into 8 portions. Shape portions into ¾-inch thick patties and dredge in panko. Place non-stick skillet over medium heat and add 1 Tbsp oil. Add dredged patties and cook 3 minutes on each side or until golden.

Prepare remoulade: Combine ¼ cup light mayonnaise, 2 tsp minced shallots, 1 tsp chopped tarragon, 1 tsp chopped parsley, 1½ tsp Dijon mustard and ¾ tsp wine vinegar. Serve remoulade with crab cakes.

<u>**Serves 4**</u>. 320 Calories per serving (2 crab cakes)

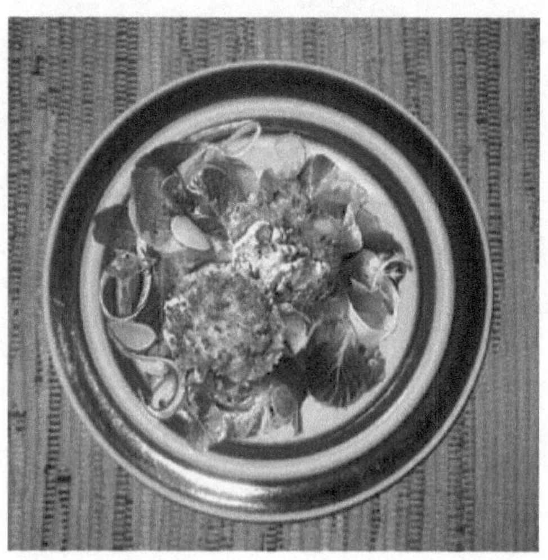

Note: Serve with a baked potato (no butter) and a large tossed salad (with 1½ tablespoons of low-calorie dressing). This adds about 170 Calories. Then the total for this meal is 490 Calories.

<u>Shrimp with Orzo</u>

   1 pound medium shrimp, peeled & deveined
   2 tablespoons olive oil, divided
   2 cloves garlic, minced
   1 onion, diced
   ½ teaspoon dried oregano
   8 ounces orzo pasta
   1 pint cherry tomatoes (about 30), halved

1. Cook orzo according to package directions. After cooked, drain and return orzo to pot; add a teaspoon of the olive oil and toss to coat. Retain orzo liquid for later use.

2.   In large skillet over medium-high heat, sauté cherry tomatoes in remaining olive oil until skin begins to crack. Stir in onion, garlic and oregano. Just before garlic turns slightly yellow add shrimp and sauté on both sides for 1 minute. Thin sauce with orzo liquid to desired consistency.

3. Plate shrimp and orzo and pour sauce over both. Add steamed Swiss chard. Serve immediately.

<u>**Serves 4.**</u>   About 400 Calories per serving

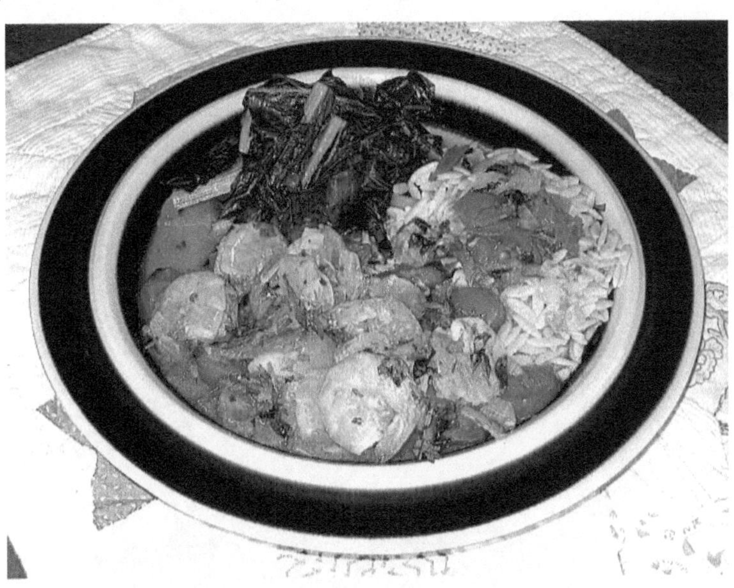

Note: There might even be room for a small (4 ounce) glass of wine. Be sure to add another 100 Calories for the wine. The total for the meal would then be 500 Calories.

Recipe 69

<u>Bay Scallops & Snow Peas</u>

    1 tablespoon olive oil
    1 large shallot, diced
    5 ounces button mushrooms, chopped coarsely
    3 ounces snow peas, halved
    ¼ teaspoon ground lemon pepper
    1 tablespoon rice vinegar
    ⅛ teaspoon (or less) red pepper flakes
    ½ pound bay scallops
    ¼ teaspoon thyme
    ¼ teaspoon tarragon

1. Heat olive oil in a skillet over medium heat. Add shallot and mushrooms. Sauté until shallot is translucent and mushrooms are cooked.
2. Stir in snow peas and remaining ingredients except scallops, thyme and tarragon. Cook for about 2 minutes.
3. Add scallops, stirring often, and cook another 3 minutes, or until scallops are white, not translucent, on all sides.
4. Stir in thyme and tarragon and cook for another thirty seconds.
5. Plate and serve.

<u>Serves 2.</u> 240 Calories per serving.

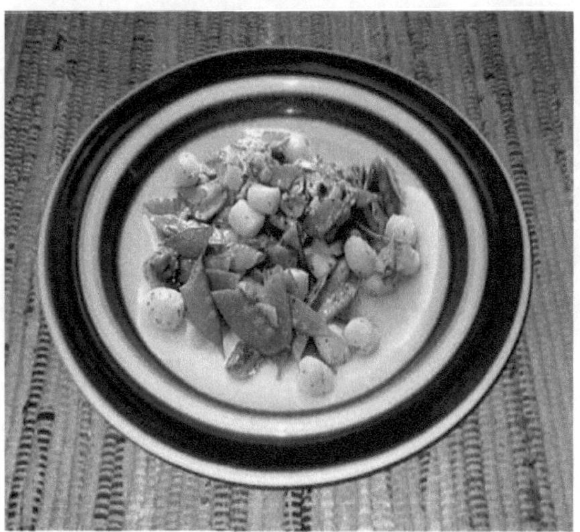

Note: The addition of a small whole-grain roll brings the total for the meal to 320 Calories. Have a small glass (4 ounces) of wine and the calorie sum is up to 420.

Recipe 70

Shrimp & Asparagus Stir Fry

    1 1/2 pounds asparagus, rinsed
    1 1/2 cups fat-skimmed chicken broth
    2 tablespoons soy sauce
    2 tablespoons cornstarch
    1/4 teaspoon white pepper
    1 tablespoon vegetable oil
    2 tablespoons minced fresh ginger
    2 cloves garlic, peeled and minced
    1 pound shelled, deveined shrimp
    12 ounces spaghetti

1) Cook pasta according to package directions
2) Meanwhile, snap tough stem ends off asparagus. Cut spears at a 45° angle into
1/2-inch-thick slices. In a small bowl, mix broth, soy sauce, cornstarch, and white pepper.
3) Set a large wok or frying pan over high heat. When hot, add oil, ginger, and garlic; stir until garlic begins to turn golden, about 30 seconds. Stir in asparagus and add 3 tablespoons water; cover and cook just until asparagus is bright green, 1 to 2 minutes. Add shrimp and stir, uncovered, until they are opaque in center of thickest part (cut to test), 2 to 3 minutes.
4) Stir broth mixture and add to pan; stir until sauce boils and thickens. Add salt to taste.
5) Set spaghetti on each of four dinner plates. Spoon shrimp and asparagus stir-fry equally over pasta.

Serves 4. 580 Calories per serving

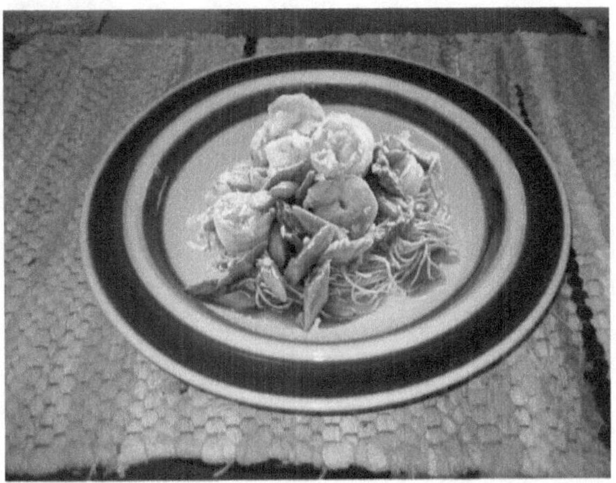

Recipe 71

Chinese Tuna Salad

    12 ounces solid white albacore tuna
    1 cup carrots, sliced
    1 cup red bell peppers, sliced
    4 green onions, diced
    1 cup edamame beans, cooked and shelled
    1 cup chow mien noodles
    2 hearts romaine lettuce
    4 cups mesclun mix or spring mix

<u>Chinese salad dressing</u>: In a jar with a tight-fitting lid combine 2 tsp garlic powder, 1 tsp dried parsley, 1 tsp dried basil, 1 tsp honey, 2 tsp soy sauce, 4 tsp sesame oil, 2 tsp Sriracha,* 4 tsp Dijon mustard, 4 tbsp olive oil, 4 tbsp rice wine vinegar and a dash of black pepper. Shake well and set aside.

In a bowl, combine romaine lettuce, mesclun mix lettuces (or spring mix), carrots, red bell pepper, green onions and edamame. Add dressing and toss. Add chow mien noodles and tuna and toss again.

Serves 4. About 445 Calories per serving.

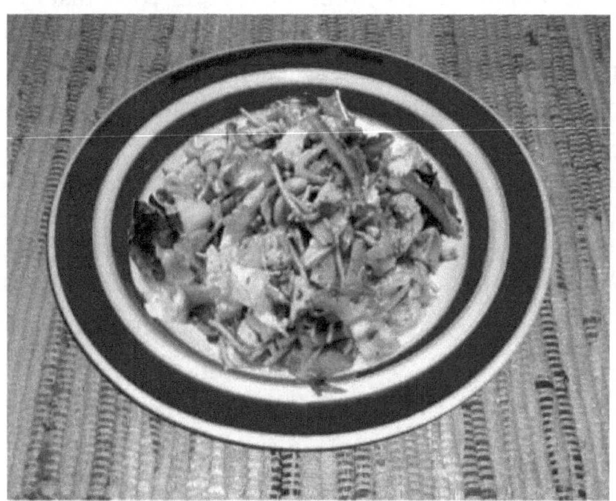

* Sriracha, is a Chinese hot sauce produced by Huy Fong Inc. (This ingredient is optional.)

Recipe 72

Penne Salad

- 2 cups uncooked penne
- 12 asparagus spears
- 12 cherry tomatoes
- 4 tablespoons extra-virgin olive oil, divided
- ½ teaspoon black pepper, divided
- 1 tablespoon minced shallots
- 2 tablespoons fresh lemon juice
- 1 tablespoon Dijon mustard
- 1 teaspoon dried herbes de Provence
- 1½ teaspoons honey
- ½ cup pitted black olives, halved
- 2 cups baby arugula
- ½ cup (2 ounces) crumbled goat cheese

1. Preheat oven to 400°F. Cook pasta according to package directions and set aside.

2. Place asparagus and tomatoes on a jelly-roll pan. Drizzle with 1 tablespoon olive oil; sprinkle with ¼ teaspoon salt and ¼ teaspoon black pepper. Toss gently to coat; arrange asparagus and tomato mixture in a single layer. Bake at 400°F for 6 minutes or until asparagus is crisp-tender.

3. Remove asparagus from pan. Place pan back in oven, and bake tomatoes an additional 4 minutes. Remove tomatoes from pan; let asparagus and tomatoes stand 10 minutes. Cut asparagus into 1-inch lengths; halve tomatoes.

4. Combine shallots and the next 4 ingredients (through honey) in a small bowl, stirring with a whisk. Gradually add remaining 3 tablespoons oil, stirring constantly with a whisk. Stir in ⅛ teaspoon salt and ¼ teaspoon black pepper.

5. Place pasta, asparagus, tomato, olives, and arugula in a large bowl; toss. Drizzle juice mixture over pasta mixture; toss. Sprinkle with cheese.

Serves 4. About 420 Calories per serving

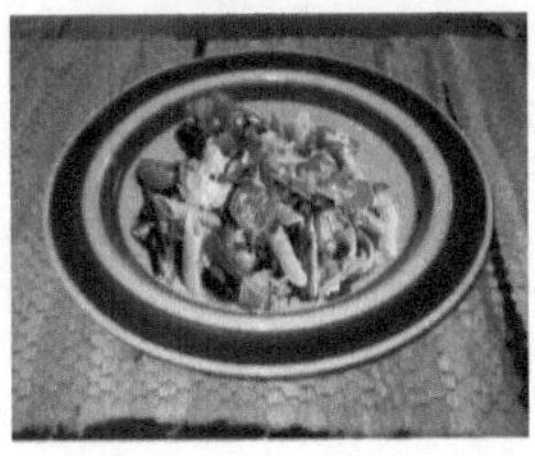

Note: Serve salad with small whole-grain roll. Then the total would be 500 Calories.

Pita Pizza

6 pita bread loaves*
¾ cup part-skim shredded mozzarella, divided
1 large red pepper, sliced
1 medium onion, sliced
6 medium mushrooms, sliced
¾ cup tomato sauce, divided
4 tablespoons olive oil

Cook olive oil in large skillet over medium-high heat. Add pepper slices, onion slices and mushroom slices and sauté until they softened.

Toast pita loaves slightly (so they don't get soggy when sauce is applied). Coat one side of pita with tomato sauce. Arrange pepper, onion and mushroom slices on individual pita loaves and sprinkle shredded mozzarella cheese on top.

In oven preheated to 400ºF, place pita loaves on baking tin coated with cooking spray. Cook approximately 5 minutes or until cheese melts. Season with salt and pepper to taste.

Serves 3. 430 Calories per serving (Two Pita Pizzas per serving.)

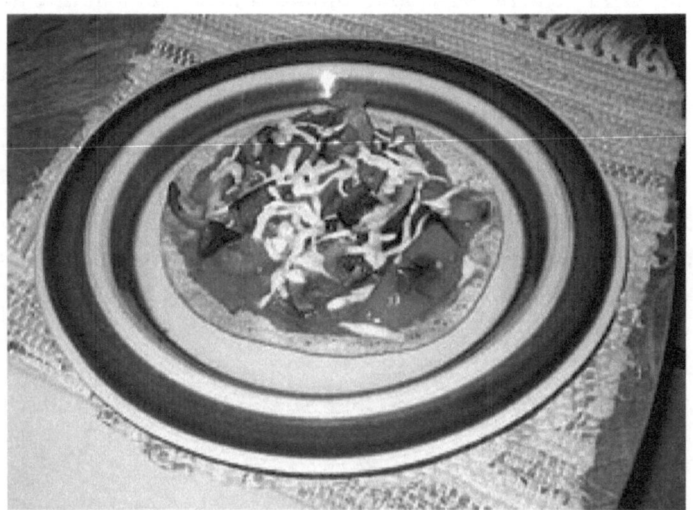

Note only one pita pizza shown. Serving size is <u>two</u> pita pizzas.

Note: Add a large tossed salad with 1½ tablespoons of low-cal dressing and the calorie total for the meal is 500.

* For example, Joseph's Flax, Oat Bran & Whole Wheat Pita Bread - 8 oz pkg.

<u>Pasta with Marinara Sauce</u>

The spiral pasta profile shown below is called fusilli, a very popular pasta shape because all those ridges hold lots of tomato sauce.

½ small onion, finely chopped
1 teaspoon olive oil
2 garlic cloves, finely chopped
1½ cups chopped plum tomatoes
½ teaspoon chopped fresh oregano
½ pound fusilli pasta
¼ teaspoon salt

Homemade Tomato sauce: Sauté chopped onion in 1 teaspoon olive oil. Add two finely chopped garlic cloves, 1½ cups chopped plum tomatoes and ½ teaspoon chopped fresh oregano. Stir and cook about 5 minutes on a low flame.

Pasta: Bring 2 quarts of lightly salted water to a boil. Add pasta and stir occasionally (to keep pasta from sticking to the bottom of the pot). Keep water boiling and cook until pasta are "al dente." (Cooking time is about 9 minutes.) Because the tomato sauce is a bit too thick, add ¼ cup of pasta liquid to the sauce to thin it. Finally drain the pasta, add the marinara sauce and serve hot.

<u>Serves 4.</u> One serving is about 250 Calories.

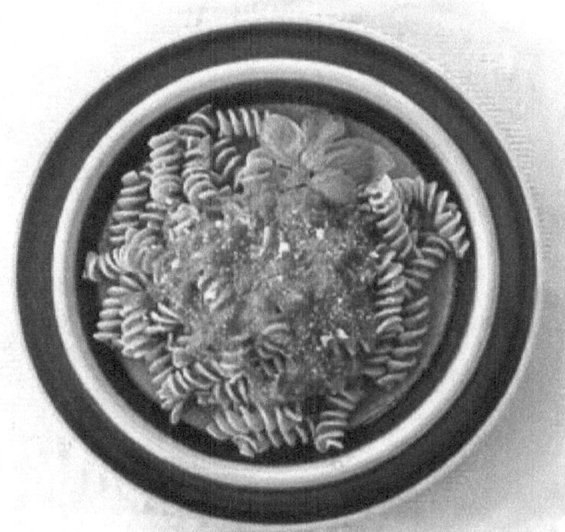

Note: We suggest the pasta be served with a small whole-grain roll and a large tossed salad (with 1½ tablespoons of low-calorie dressing). This adds about 150 Calories to the meal. Then the total would be 450 Calories. (There might even be room for a small glass of red wine. Be sure to add another 25 Calories per ounce for the wine.)

Recipe 75

Quick Pasta alla Puttanesca

This famous pasta dish originated in Naples Italy. Puttanesca means "ladies of the night." Although the exact origin of the meal is unclear, one thing is clear: It's delicious! Here is one of many recipe versions.

   ½ pound spaghetti
   20 black or green pitted olives
   14.5-oz can diced tomatoes
   4 oz tomato sauce
   2 tablespoon extra-virgin olive oil
   3 cloves of garlic, chopped
   1 tablespoon dried minced onion
   ½ teaspoon crushed red pepper flakes
   1 tablespoon capers drained and rinsed
   ¼ cup currants

Cook spaghetti according to package directions. Drain and return spaghetti to pot; add a teaspoon extra-virgin olive oil and toss to coat.

Heat remaining olive oil in large skillet over medium-high heat. Add red pepper flakes; cook and stir 1 to 2 minutes or until sizzling. Add onion and garlic; cook and stir 1 minute. Add canned tomatoes with juice, tomato sauce, olives, currants and capers. Cook over medium-high heat, stirring frequently, until sauce is heated through.

Serves 4. About 345 Calories per serving

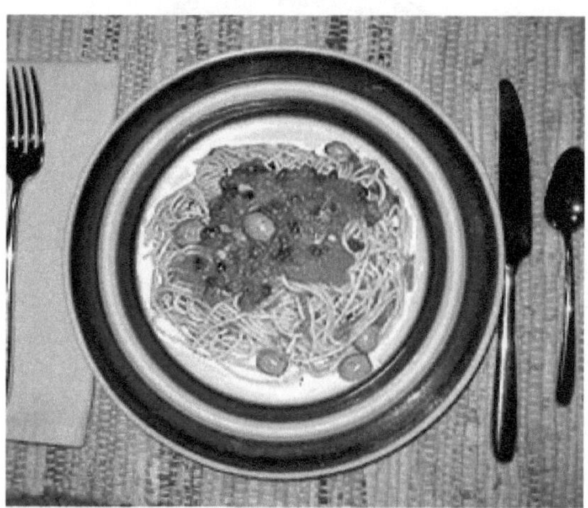

Note: We suggest the pasta be served with a small whole-grain roll and a large tossed salad (with 1½ tablespoons of low-calorie dressing). This adds about 150 Calories to the meal. This adds about 150 Calories to the meal. Then the total for this meal would be 495 Calories.

Recipe 76

Fettuccine in Summer Sauce

This sauce is often served in the summer because it's lighter than what is usually dished up with pasta. But despite its name the sauce is wonderful year round.

  ½ lb fettuccine pasta
  8 oz fresh asparagus, trimmed & cut in 2-inch pieces
  ¾ pint cherry tomatoes (about 20), halved
  2 Tbsp plus 1 tsp extra-virgin olive oil, divided
  2 cloves of garlic, chopped
  ½ small onion, diced

Cook fettuccine according to package directions. Drain and return pasta to pot; add a teaspoon of the olive oil and toss to coat. Meanwhile steam asparagus and drain.

In large skillet over medium-high heat, sauté cherry tomatoes in remaining 2 tablespoons of olive oil until skin begins to crack. Add onion and cook until translucent. Stir in garlic. Thin sauce with pasta liquid to desired consistency. Toss cooked pasta and asparagus into sauce and serve immediately.

Serves 4. About 290 Calories per serving

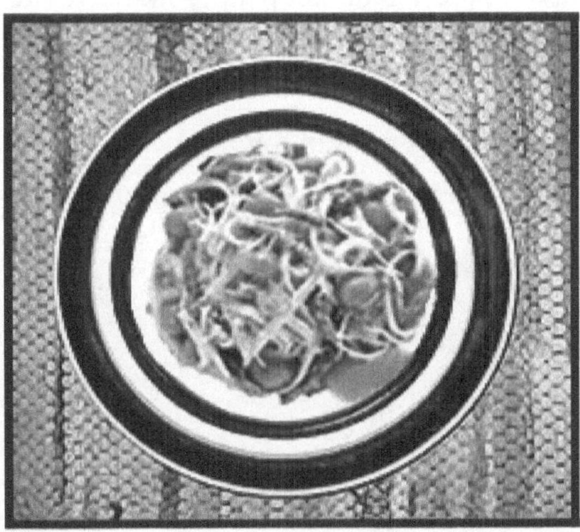

Note: We suggest the pasta be served with a small whole-grain roll and a large tossed salad (with 1½ tablespoons of low-calorie dressing). Then the total for this meal would be 440 Calories.

Recipe 77

<u>Pasta Rapini</u>

   2 cloves garlic - coarsely chopped
   1½ cups of crushed San Marzano tomatoes
   2 cups Rapini (broccoli rabe)
   1 tablespoon crushed red pepper flakes (optional)
   ½ pound medium-sized spaghetti

<u>Tomato Sauce:</u> In large pan, sauté two tablespoons olive oil over medium-high heat. Add the garlic and sauté until translucent (but not browned). Add crushed San Marzano tomatoes (use plum tomatoes if San Marzano are not available) and bring to a boil. Reduce heat to low and simmer for about 30 minutes or until cooked. Season with salt and pepper. Set aside.

<u>Rapini:</u> Discard the tough stems and slice into 2-inch pieces. Bring a pot of water to a boil. Add Rapini (a variety of the vegetable broccoli rabe) and 1 tablespoon salt. Blanch Rapini about 5 minutes or until slightly cooked but still crunchy at stems. Drain, set aside and cover.

Cook pasta according to package instructions until al dente. Three minutes before pasta is ready, add the Rapini to the sauté pan (containing the tomato sauce). Heat mixture over medium heat. Drain pasta and add it to the pan with the Rapini and tomatoes. Add hot pepper flakes (optional) and toss for 1 to 2 minutes over high heat. Drizzle lightly with extra virgin olive oil and plate. Delicious!

Serves 4. About 290 Calories per serving

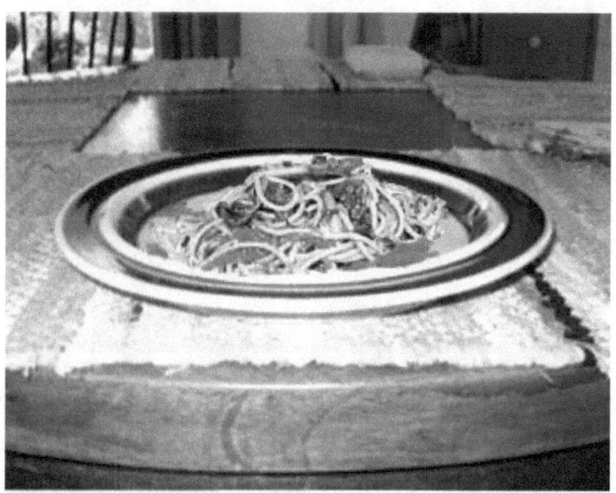

Note: Serve the pasta with a small whole-grain roll and a large tossed salad (with 1½ tablespoons of low-calorie dressing). Then the total for this meal would be 440 Calories.

Recipe 78

Pasta e Fagioli

This is one variation of a traditional, nutritious peasant dish served all over
Italy.

    14.5-oz can whole tomatoes with juice, crushed
    14.5-oz can cannellini beans, drained*
    1 cup of any tube-shaped pasta
    2 tablespoon olive oil
    1 medium onion, diced
    2 cloves garlic, minced
    1 stalk celery, finely chopped
    3 cups vegetable stock
    2 cups fresh baby spinach or escarole
    1 tsp dried basil
    ½ teaspoon dried oregano
    2 Tbsp fresh parsley, chopped

Heat olive oil, onion and celery in large saucepan over medium heat. Sauté
until onions are golden brown. Add garlic and stir constantly for one minute.
Pour in tomatoes and their juices and bring to a boil. Add beans and chicken
stock and return to a boil. Stir in spinach (or escarole) and seasonings.
Simmer for about 5 minutes. Add pasta and cook about 15 minutes or until
pasta is tender but firm. If needed, thin soup with hot water.

Ladle into soup bowls. Garnish with grated Parmesan cheese. Salt and
pepper to taste.

Serves 4. About 300 Calories per serving.

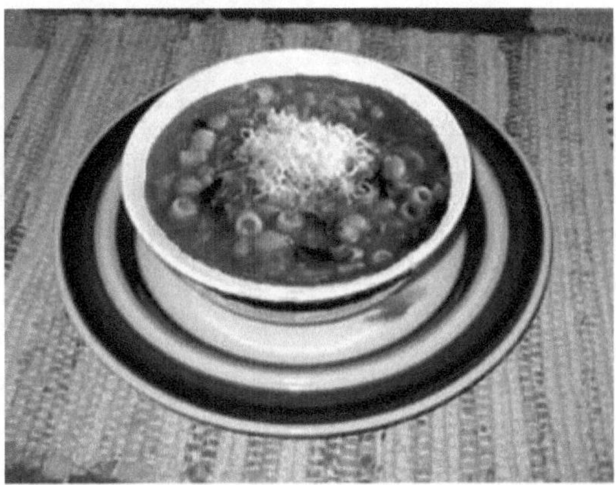

Note: We suggest the pasta be served with a small whole-grain roll and a
large tossed salad (with 1½ tablespoons of low-calorie dressing). Then the
total for this meal would be 440 Calories.

<u>Healthy Pasta Salad</u>

- ½ pound fusilli pasta, cooked until tender but firm
- 2 broccoli crowns, chopped
- ¼ pint cherry tomatoes (about 8), halved
- ½ cup black olives, halved
- ½ cup garbanzo beans (chick peas)
- ½ cup fresh light mozzarella cheese, chopped
- 1 tablespoon basil
- 1 tablespoon rosemary
- 2 teaspoons garlic powder
- ¼ cup of low-calorie dressing

Combine dry ingredients in a medium-size bowl. Stir in salad dressing. Mix thoroughly. Salt and black pepper to taste.

<u>**Serves 4**</u>. 370 Calories per serving.

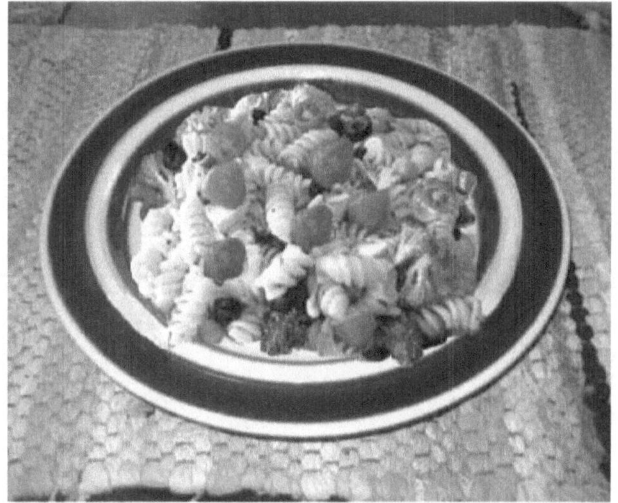

Note: Serve the pasta with a small whole-grain roll and a large tossed salad (with 1½ tablespoons of low-calorie dressing). Then the total for this meal would be 520 Calories.

Recipe 80

<u>Pasta Pomodoro</u>

Pasta Pomodoro (Italian for pasta with tomatoes) is typically prepared with angel hair pasta, olive oil, fresh tomatoes, and fresh basil. It's light, delicious and easy to make.

¾	pound angel hair pasta
1½	pints cherry tomatoes (about 45), halved
8	fresh basil leaves, chopped
4	cloves garlic, minced
2	tablespoons olive oil
4	Tbsp grated parmesan cheese

Cook angel hair pasta per package directions. Over medium heat, sauté the garlic in olive oil until it just starts to turn golden. Add tomatoes and cook for about 10 minutes, or until they just start to release juices. Turn off the heat and stir basil into the sauce. Over the cooked pasta, spoon the tomato sauce with a little of the pasta water and garnish with more basil and grated cheese.

<u>Serves 4</u>. 420 Calories per serving

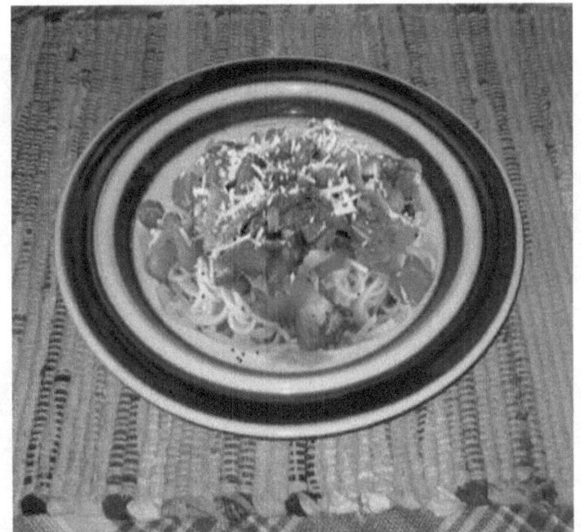

Above prepared with mix of cherry and plum tomatoes.

Note: Serve the pasta with a small whole-grain roll and a large tossed salad (with 1½ tablespoons of low-calorie dressing). This adds about 150 Calories to the meal. Then the total for this serving would be 570 Calories.

Recipe 81

Pasta Primavera

- ¾ pound penne pasta
- 2 cups broccoli florets
- 1 red bell pepper, sliced
- 1 carrot, cut to 1-inch sticks
- ½ cup frozen green peas & ½ cup frozen sweet corn
- 1 small onion, chopped
- 1 tablespoon minced garlic
- 3 tablespoons olive oil
- 1 teaspoon fresh basil, chopped

Cook penne pasta per package directions. Drain and place pasta in a bowl. Pre-cook the carrot and broccoli florets.

In a large heavy skillet, heat the olive oil and sauté onion and garlic until lightly golden. Add vegetables and sauté until the peppers are soft. Combine sautéed vegetables in the bowl with the pasta. Toss well. Garnish with chopped basil, season to taste, and top with freshly grated Parmesan cheese.

Serves 4. 460 Calories per serving

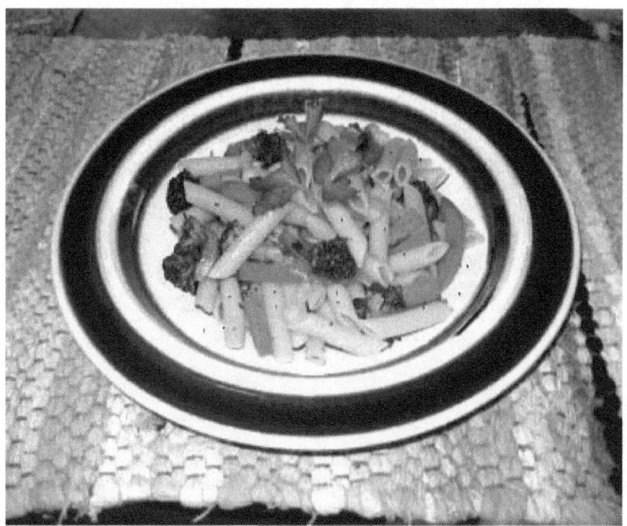

Photo taken before grated cheese was added.

<h1 style="text-align:center">Recipe 82</h1>

<u>Pasta with Veggies</u>

- ½ pound fusilli pasta
- 2 small yellow squash, halved and cut into ½-inch-thick slices
- 1 medium orange bell pepper, cut into 1-inch pieces
- 8 oz. small broccoli florets (3 cups)
- 2 cups halved cherry tomatoes
- 8 green onions, thinly sliced (½ cup)
- 3 Tbs. olive oil
- 3 cloves garlic, minced (about 1 Tbsp)
- ½ cup torn fresh basil leaves
- 1 tsp. grated lemon zest

Combine oil, garlic, and lemon zest in small bowl. Set aside. Cook pasta in large pot of boiling, salted water according to package directions.   Add squash and bell pepper 4 minutes before end of cooking time. Add broccoli 3 minutes before end of cooking time. Drain pasta and vegetables, reserving ½ cup cooking water.

Return pasta mixture to pot, and stir in tomatoes, green onions, basil, oil mixture, and reserved cooking water. Heat over medium-low heat until tomatoes are hot. Serve with Parmesan cheese, if desired.

<u>**Serves 4**</u>. 350 Calories per serving

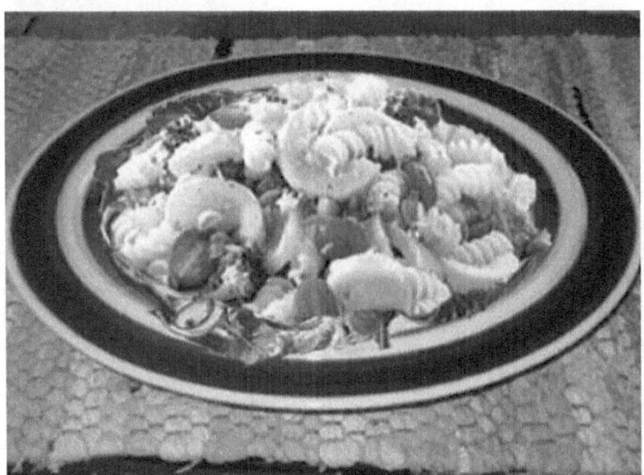

Photo shows two servings of pasta.

Note: Serve with a large tossed salad (with 1½ tablespoons of low-calorie dressing) and a small whole-grain roll. This adds about 150 Calories. Then the total for this meal is 400 Calories.

Recipe 83

<u>Easy Penne Pasta</u>

    1 16-ounce box penne pasta
    1 tablespoon olive oil
    ¼ teaspoon red pepper flakes
    1 24-ounce jar tomato basil sauce
    ½ cup Parmesan cheese, grated
    ½ cup Italian parsley leaves, chopped

1. Bring a large pot of lightly salted water to a boil.
2. Meanwhile heat tomato-basil sauce and stir in red pepper flakes.
3. Cook the pasta according to package directions, drain and toss with tomato sauce. If desired, thin sauce with pasta water. Stir in olive oil before serving.
4. Sprinkle each serving with Parmesan cheese, parsley and salt to taste.

<u>**Serves 6.**</u> About 375 Calories per serving

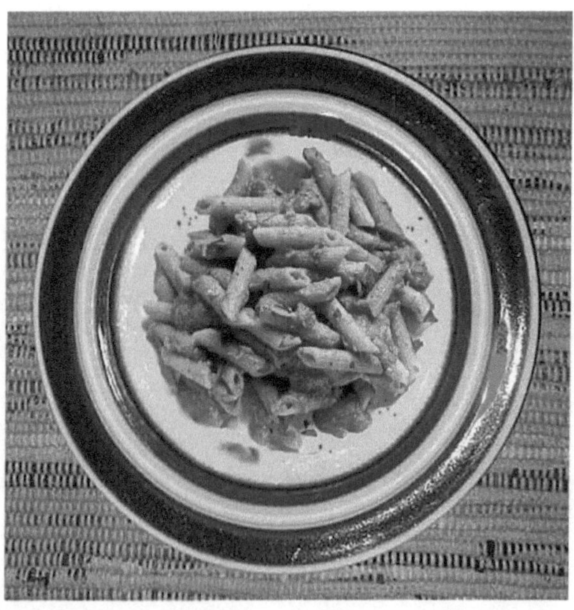

Note: Serve the pasta with a small whole-grain roll and a large tossed salad (with 1½ tablespoons of low-calorie dressing). This adds about 150 Calories to the meal. Then the total for this serving would be about 525 Calories.

Recipe 84

<u>Low-Cal Eggplant Parmesan</u>

  3 medium eggplants, cut crosswise into ½-inch slices
  3 tablespoons olive oil
  1 large onion, finely chopped
  1 large clove garlic, thinly sliced
  1½ teaspoons dried oregano
  1 28-ounce can plum or crushed tomatoes
  1 tablespoon red wine vinegar
  ½ cup (packed) fresh basil leaves
  ½ cup freshly grated Parmesan cheese
  ⅓ cup fine dry bread crumbs

1. Preheat oven to 450°F. Brush both sides eggplant slices with olive oil, and place in single layer on baking sheets. Bake until undersides are golden brown, 10 to 15 minutes. Then turn and bake until other side is lightly browned. Set aside. Reduce oven to 375°F.

2. Meanwhile, in large saucepan over medium heat, add 2 tablespoons olive oil, onion, oregano and garlic. Sauté until soft, about 10 minutes. Add plum tomatoes and their juices. Break up whole tomatoes. Cover, reduce heat to low and simmer 15 to 20 minutes.

3. Add vinegar, basil and salt and pepper to taste. In a 10-by-6-inch baking pan, spoon a small amount of tomato sauce, then add a thin scattering of parmesan cheese, then a single layer of eggplant. Repeat until all ingredients are used, ending with a little sauce and a sprinkling of parmesan cheese. In a small bowl, combine bread crumbs with enough olive oil to moisten. Sprinkle on top.

4. Bake until eggplant mixture is bubbly and center is hot, 30 to 45 minutes depending on size of pan and thickness of layers. Remove from heat and allow to rest before serving.

<u>Serves 5.</u>   About 270 Calories per serving

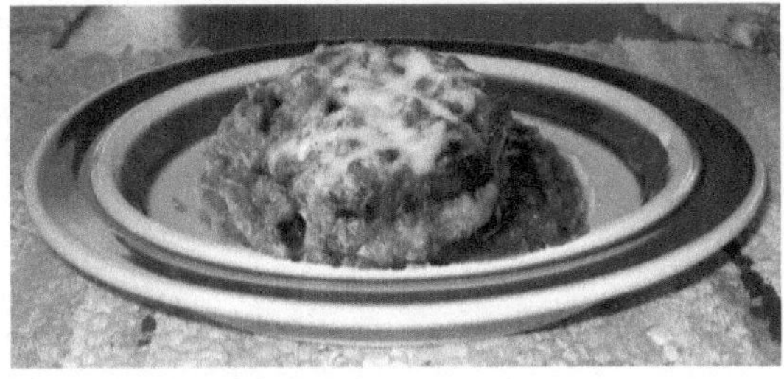

Note: Serve with a small whole-grain roll and a large tossed salad (with 1½ tablespoons of low-calorie dressing). Then the total for this serving would be about 420 Calories.

Recipe 85

<u>Tortellini Pasta & Beans</u>

1 9-ounce refrigerated package cheese-filled spinach tortellini
1 15-ounce can cannellini (white kidney) beans, rinsed and drained
¾ cup crumbled garlic-and-herb-flavored feta cheese (3 ounces)
2 tablespoons olive oil
1 large tomato, chopped
4 cups baby spinach

1) Cook tortellini according to package directions. Drain and return to pan.
2) Add drained beans, feta cheese, and olive oil to tortellini in saucepan.
Cook over medium heat until beans are hot and cheese begins to melt, gently
stirring occasionally. Add tomato; cook another minute. Sprinkle black
pepper.
3) Divide spinach among four dinner plates. Top with tortellini mixture.

<u>Serves 4</u>. 450 Calories per serving

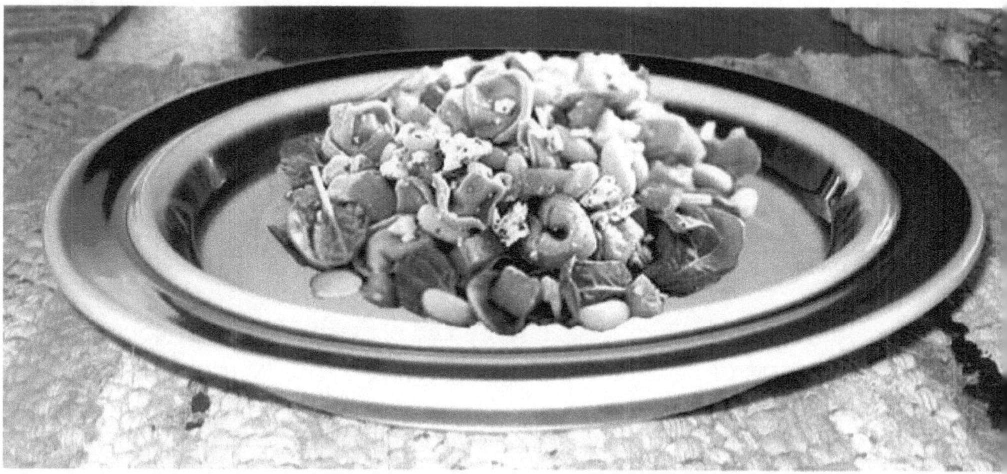

Note: Add a small whole-grain roll and the total for this dish would be about
530 Calories per serving.

Recipe 86

<u>Pasta with Cheese & Walnuts</u>

- ½ cup walnuts
- 2 cloves garlic
- 1 tablespoon olive
- 1 box medium whole-wheat shells
- 1 pound frozen peas
- 6 ounces goat cheese

1) Heat covered 6-quart pot of water to boiling on high. Add 2 teaspoons salt.

2) In an 8- to 10-inch skillet, combine walnuts, garlic, and oil. Cook on medium until golden and fragrant, stirring occasionally. Stir in ⅛ teaspoon each salt and freshly ground black pepper.

3) Add pasta to boiling water in pot. Cook 1 minute less than minimum time that label directs, stirring occasionally. Add peas; cook 1 minute longer. Reserve 1 cup pasta cooking water. Drain pasta and peas; return to pot.

4) Add goat cheese, ½ cooking water, ¼ teaspoon salt, and ½ teaspoon freshly ground black pepper. If mixture is dry, toss with additional cooking water.

5) To serve, top with garlic-and-walnut mixture.

<u>Serves 4</u>. 490 Calories per serving

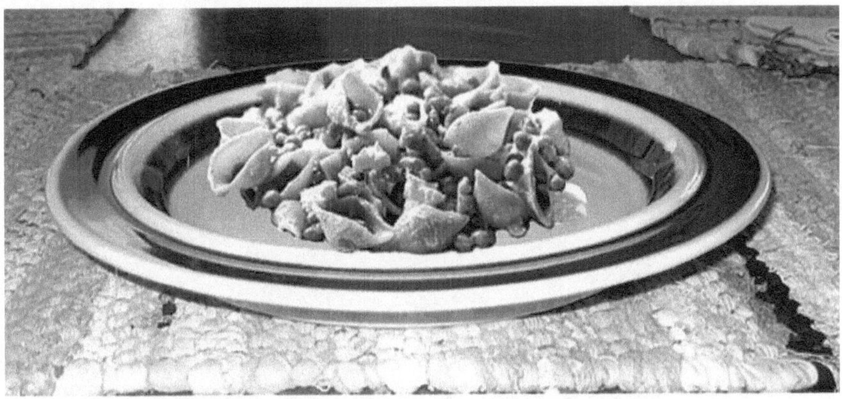

Note: The addition of a large tossed salad with 1½ tablespoons of low-cal dressing brings the calorie total to 560 per serving.

Grandma's Pizza

The following is a pizza recipe used by Gail Johnson's Italian grandmother. She was from a small mountain village located between Rome and Naples.

Pizza dough: To save time use prepared dough. To start, flour a large cutting board. Divide one pound of prepared pizza dough into four parts. Roll out each dough ball as thin as possible.

Tomato sauce: Sauté ½ small onion, chopped fine, in 1 teaspoon olive oil. Add two finely chopped garlic cloves, 1½ cups chopped plum tomatoes and ½ teaspoon chopped fresh oregano. Stir and cook about 5 minutes on a low flame.

Pizza preparation & cooking: On each pizza, spread evenly ¼ cup of tomato sauce. Add ½ ounce of shredded part-skim mozzarella cheese, 1 teaspoon Parmesan cheese, 3 slices of a Portobello mushroom, some torn fresh basil, and drizzle with extra-virgin olive oil. Put pizzas on a pan and place in 475 °F oven for about 15 to 20 minutes, or until crust is crisp and cheese is just melting. (Freeze left over sauce for another day.)

<u>Serves 4</u>. Each pizza contains approximately 350 Calories.

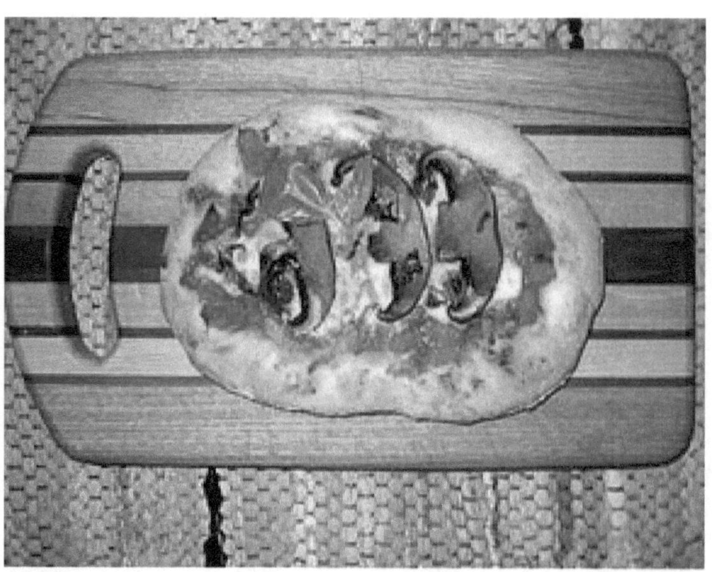

Note: Serve the pizza with a large tossed salad (with 1½ tablespoons of low-calorie dressing). This adds about 70 Calories. Then the total for this meal would be 420 Calories.

Recipe 88

Penne with Eggplant & Tomato

    3 tablespoons olive oil
    2 celery stalks, sliced
    1 eggplant, cut into ½-inch pieces
    1 pint grape tomatoes, halved
    ¼ cup tomato paste
    ¼ cup white wine vinegar
    1 tablespoon sugar
    2 tablespoons capers
    1 cup fresh parsley, chopped
    ¾ pound penne pasta

1) Cook penne according to package directions.
2) Meanwhile, heat 2 tablespoons of oil in a large saucepan over medium-high heat. Add celery and cook for 3 minutes. Stir in eggplant and tomatoes.
3) In a small bowl, combine the tomato paste, vinegar, ¼ cup water, 2 teaspoons salt,
¼ teaspoon pepper, and the sugar. Stir into eggplant mixture.
4) Cover and reduce heat to medium-low. Cook, stirring occasionally, until eggplant
is tender, 15 to 20 minutes. Remove from heat and stir in capers and parsley.
5) Toss with remaining oil; let cool. Combine with eggplant mixture and serve.

Serves 4. About 450 Calories per serving.

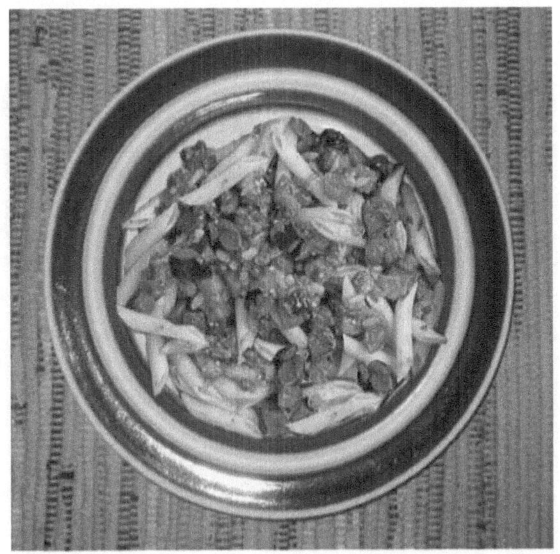

Recipe 89

Pasta & Beans with Escarole

    12 ounces carrots, cut to 1/2" thick coins
    2 stalks celery, cut to 1/2" thick slices
    2 onions, chopped
    2 cloves garlic, chopped
    3 tablespoons olive oil
    2 15-ounce cans chopped tomatoes
    3 cups black eyed peas
    2 bay leaves
    1 pound escarole, tear into bite-size pieces
    4 ounces pasta of your choice

1) Cook pasta according to package directions.

2) Meanwhile, heat 1 tablespoon olive oil in large pot over medium heat. When hot, add carrots, celery, onion and a pinch of salt and cook, stirring occasionally, until vegetables begin to soften, 5 to 7 minutes.

3) Add garlic and cook, stirring until fragrant, about 1 minute. Add tomatoes, peas, bay leaves and 5 cups water. Bring to a boil, then lower the heat so the mixture bubbles steadily. Cook, stirring occasionally, until tomatoes start to break down, 10 to 15 minutes.

4) Remove bay leaves and add escarole and pasta. Adjust heat so liquid is at steady bubble; cook, stirring occasionally and adding water until mixture achieves desired consistency.

5) When pasta is just tender and escarole has softened, divide between 4 bowls and drizzle with the remaining 1 tablespoon olive oil.

Serves 4. Approximately 450 Calories per serving.

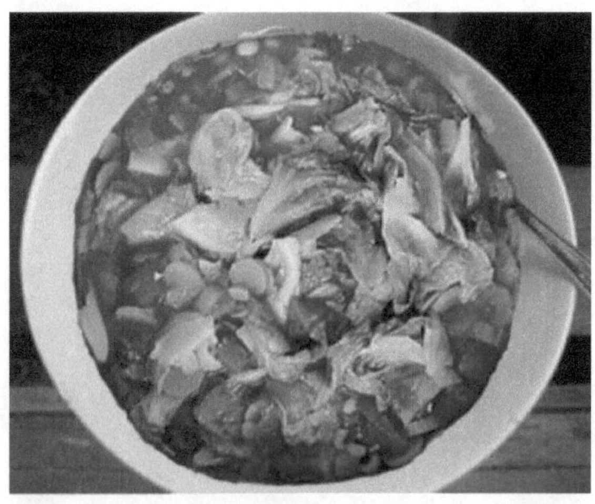

Recipe 90

<u>Pasta with Pesto</u>

Simple recipe and simply delicious!

   1 16 ounce package of pasta*
   ½ cup chopped onion
   2   tablespoons pesto
   2   tablespoons olive oil
   2   tablespoons grated Parmesan cheese

1) Cook pasta according to package directions.
2) Meanwhile, prepare pesto mixture: Heat olive oil in a frying pan over medium heat. When hot, add onion, salt and pepper. Cook until onions are soft, about 5 minutes.
3) In a large bowl, mix pesto mixture into pasta. Sir in grated cheese. Serve.

<u>Serves 4</u>. About 450 Calories per serving.

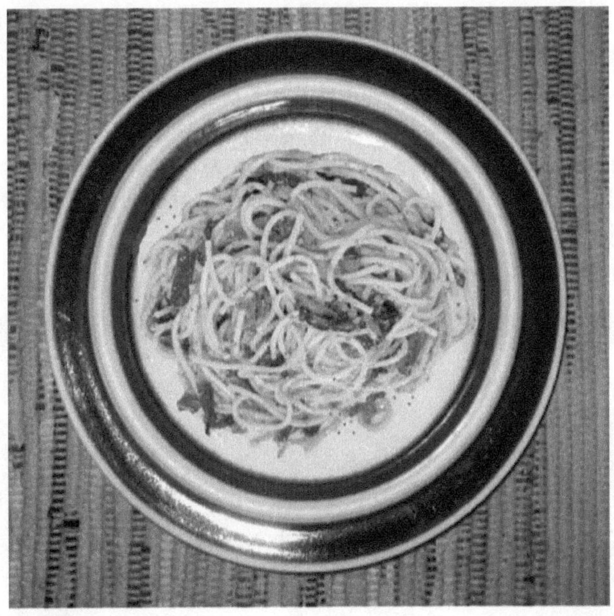

* Use any type of pasta.

Recipe 91

<u>Pasta with Cherry Tomatoes & Spinach</u>

  2 cups uncooked penne pasta
  2 teaspoons olive oil
  ¼ teaspoon crushed red pepper
  1 large garlic clove, thinly sliced
  2 cups cherry tomatoes, halved
  ¼ cup vegetable broth
  10 Kalamata olives, pitted and coarsely chopped
  4 cups baby spinach
  ¼ cup torn basil leaves
  4 tablespoons Parmesan cheese, grated

1) Cook pasta according to package directions. Reserve ½ cup cooking liquid.
2) Meanwhile, heat a large skillet over medium heat. Add oil and swirl to coat. Add red pepper and garlic; sauté 30 seconds. Add tomatoes, broth, ¼ teaspoon salt, ¼ teaspoon black pepper and olives; cook about 6 minutes or until tomatoes begin to break down, stirring occasionally.
3) Add pasta and reserved pasta cooking liquid to pan; simmer 2 minutes. Stir in spinach and basil; cook 2 minutes or until greens wilt.
4) Divide pasta mixture evenly among 4 bowls; top with Parmesan cheese and serve while hot.
<u>Serves 4</u>. About 320 Calories per serving.

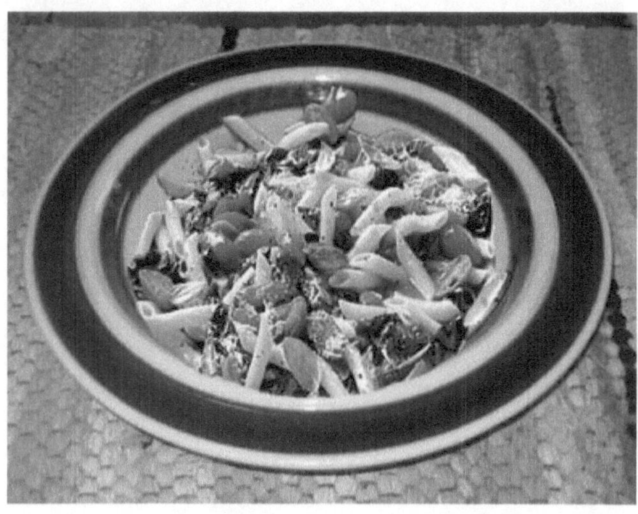

Recipe 92

<u>Pasta with Eggplant & Zucchini</u>

3 tablespoons olive oil
2 cloves garlic, chopped
1 28-ounce can crushed tomatoes
4 tablespoons fresh parsley, chopped
2 tablespoons dried oregano
⅛ teaspoon red pepper flakes
1 pound eggplant, chopped into 1-inch cubes
½ pound zucchini, cut into 1-inch slices
¾ pound penne pasta
¼ cup Parmesan cheese, grated

1) Prepare sauce: Add 1 tablespoon of oil into a saucepan over medium heat. Add garlic, and cook for a minute or so, until fragrant. Add tomatoes and sprinkle in parsley, oregano, red pepper flakes, and a pinch of salt and pepper. Bring to a boil, then reduce to a simmer. Stir occasionally for about 15 minutes.
2) Pour remainder of oil into a large skillet set over medium-high heat. Add eggplant, zucchini and a pinch of salt and pepper. Cook until both are slightly browned and tender, about 15 minutes.
3) Add the eggplant and zucchini to the saucepan and cook for another 15 minutes.
4) Cook the pasta according to package instructions. Plate pasta, and then top with tomato sauce. Sprinkle a little grated cheese on top.

<u>Serves 4</u>. About 350 Calories per serving.

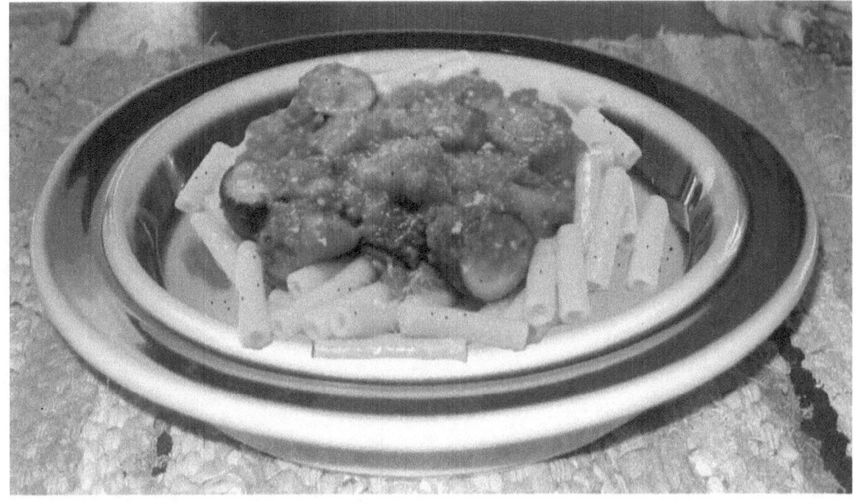

Recipe 93

<u>**Linguine in Clam Sauce**</u>

  2 tablespoons olive oil
  2 cloves garlic, chopped
  2 3-ounce cans clams, drained and chopped
  1 8-ounce bottle clam juice
  2 tablespoons fresh parsley, chopped
  ½ pound linguine
  2 tablespoons Parmesan cheese, grated

1) Cook pasta according to package directions. Reserve ½ cup pasta water.
2) Sauté over medium heat chopped garlic in olive oil until garlic is golden, about 1 minute. Add in clams, clam juice, and ½ cup pasta water. Reduce heat and simmer until sauce has
been reduced in half.
3) Plate linguine. Pour sauce over pasta and sprinkle with grated cheese and parsley.

<u>**Serves 4**</u>. About 450 Calories per serving.

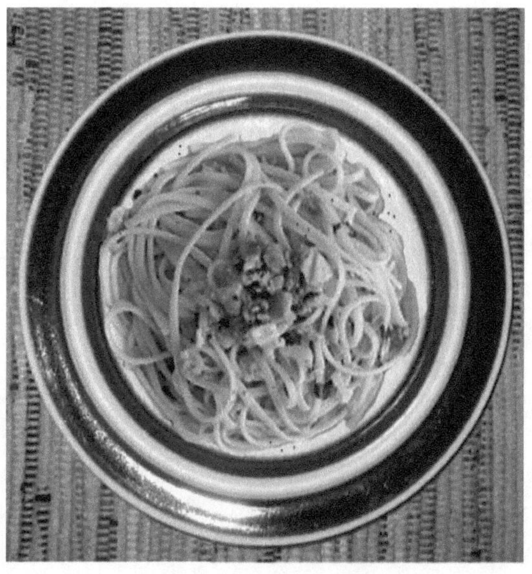

<u>Penne with Kale & Sun-dried Tomatoes</u>

    2 tablespoons olive oil
    2 cloves garlic, chopped
    1 pound kale, roughly chopped w/o stems
    ½ cup sun-dried tomatoes
    ½ cup vegetable stock
    ¾ pound penne 840+420
    2 tablespoons Parmesan cheese, grated

1) Cook pasta according to package directions. Reserve ½ cup pasta water.
2) In a large skillet, sauté over medium heat chopped garlic in olive oil until garlic is golden, about 1 minute. Add in kale, sun-dried tomatoes and vegetable stock. Cook until kale has wilted.
3) Toss in penne. Add some or all pasta water if desired.
4) Plate and sprinkle Parmesan cheese.

<u>Serves 4</u>. About 430 Calories per serving.

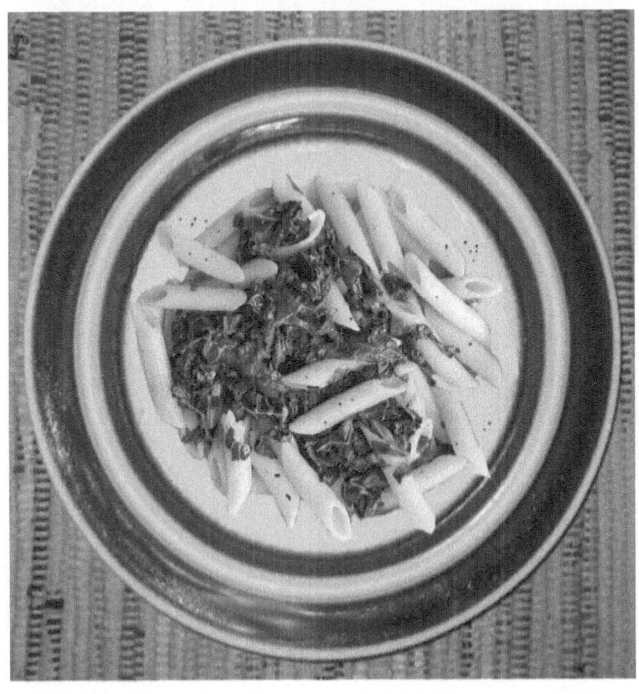

Recipe 95

<u>Beans & Greens Salad</u>

    ⅓ cup chopped oregano
    ⅓ cup chopped parsley
    3 cloves garlic, chopped
    1 lemon, juiced

Prepare dressing by combining above ingredients and stirring in ¼ cup extra-virgin olive oil. Salt and black pepper to taste.

    ½ pound mesclun mix
    ¼ pound green beans
    19-oz can garbanzo beans (chickpeas)

Arrange mesclun mix, garbanzo beans and green beans on large platter. Drizzle dressing over salad.

<u>Serves 4</u>. Approximately 260 Calories per serving.

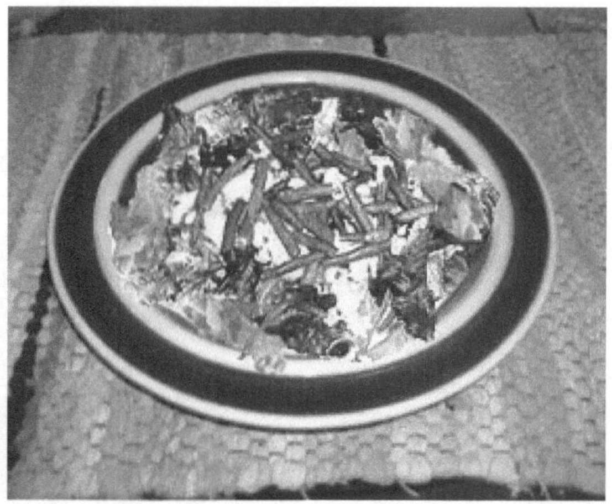

Note: We suggest the beans and greens salad be served with a small whole-grain roll. The total for this meal would be 330 Calories.

<u>Four-Bean Plus Salad</u>

Note that the total caloric value of the salad will change very little, if the proportions of the bean varieties and corn are varied – according to taste.

½ cup canned red kidney beans, drained & rinsed
½ cup canned black beans, drained & rinsed
½ cup canned chick peas, drained & rinsed
½ cup canned cannelloni beans, drained & rinsed
½ cup canned corn, drained
1 small red pepper, chopped
1 small green pepper, chopped
2 tablespoons extra-virgin olive oil
2 tablespoons lemon juice

In a large bowl mix red kidney beans, black beans, chick peas, cannelloni beans, corn and chopped red and green peppers. Stir in olive oil and lemon juice and plate.

<u>**Serves about 6**</u>. One serving is ½ cup – with about 135 Calories per serving

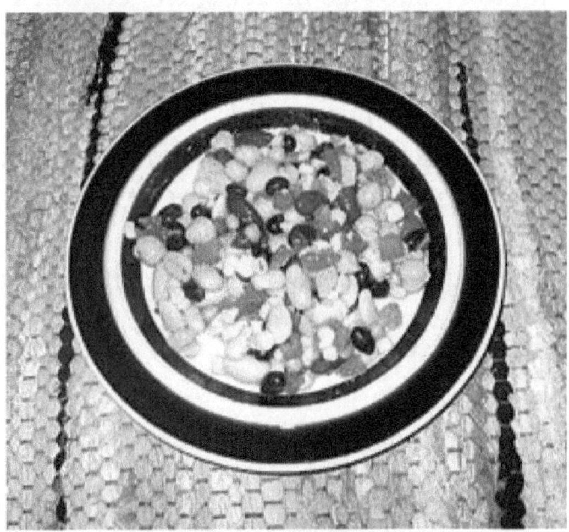

Note: We suggest this salad be served with a broiled white fish (6 oz) and a large tossed salad (with 1½ tablespoons of low-calorie dressing). This adds about 320 Calories to the meal. Then the total for this meal would be 455 Calories.

Recipe 97

<u>Tomato Risotto Salad</u>

   1 bag microwave-in-bag green beans
   1¾ cups vegetable broth
   2 tablespoons butter
   1 small onion
   2 cups Arborio rice
   2 pounds ripe tomatoes
   2 cups fresh corn kernels
   2 ounces grated Parmesan cheese
   2 tablespoons chopped basil

1) Cook green beans according to package directions. Cut into 1-inch. pieces.

2) In 2-quart saucepan, heat broth and 2 cups water to boiling. While broth mixture heats, in 4-quart bowl, microwave butter and onion, uncovered, on high for 3 minutes or until softened. Stir in rice and cook another minute.

3) Stir broth-water mixture into rice mixture. Cover with vented plastic wrap; microwave on medium (50% power) about 10 minutes.

4) Meanwhile, in food processor, puree half of tomatoes; strain juice through sieve into measuring cup, pressing on solids. Discard solids and chop remaining tomatoes. Stir 1½cups tomato juice into rice mixture. Cover with vented plastic wrap and microwave on Medium heat 5 minutes or until liquid is absorbed.

5) Stir corn into rice mixture. Cover with vented plastic wrap; microwave on Medium 3 minutes or until corn is heated through. Stir Parmesan cheese, green beans, tomatoes, half of basil, ½ teaspoon salt, and ¼ teaspoon pepper into rice mixture (the risotto). Sprinkle with basil.

<u>Serves 6</u>. 370 Calories per serving.

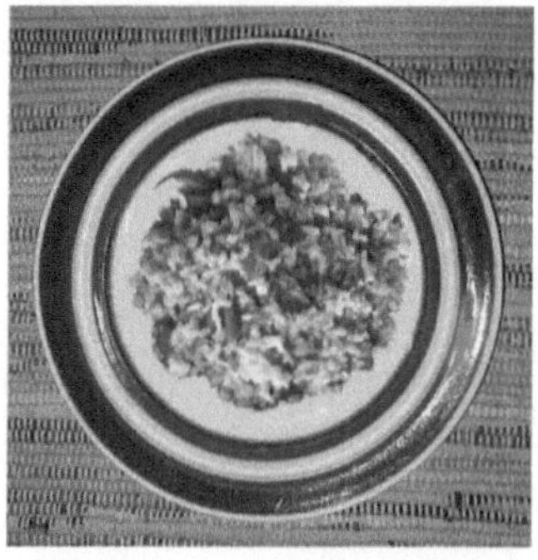

Note: Serve this salad with a small whole-grain roll. This adds about 80 Calories. Then the total for the meal would be 450 Calories.

Recipe 98

<u>Quinoa with Veggies Salad</u>

1 cup water
½ cup uncooked quinoa
¾ cup fresh parsley leaves
½ cup thinly sliced celery
½ cup thinly sliced green onions
½ cup finely chopped dried apricots
3 tablespoons fresh lemon juice
1 tablespoon olive oil
1 tablespoon raw honey
¼ teaspoon salt
¼ teaspoon black pepper
¼ cup unsalted pumpkin seed kernels, toasted

1. Bring water and quinoa to a boil in a medium saucepan. Cover, reduce heat, and simmer 20 minutes or until liquid is absorbed.
2. Spoon into a bowl and fluff with a fork. Add parsley, celery, onions, and apricots.
3. Whisk lemon juice, olive oil, honey, salt, and black pepper. Add to quinoa mixture, and toss well. Top with pumpkin seeds. Serve at room temperature.

<u>**Serves 4.**</u> 240 Calories per serving

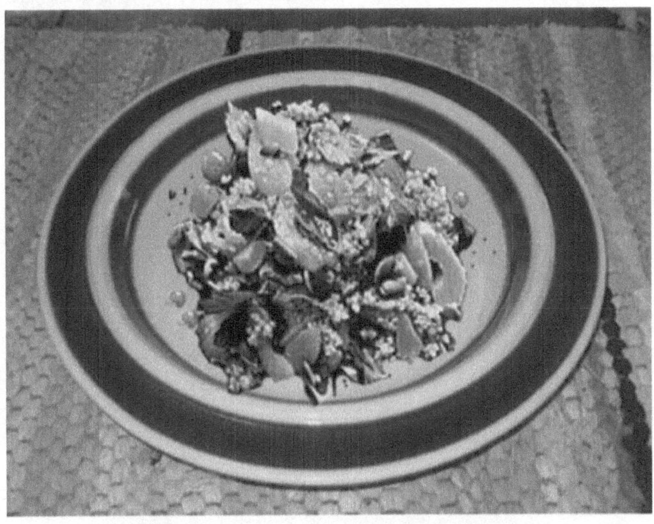

Note: Add a small whole-grain roll which brings the total for the meal to 320 Calories. Have a small glass (4 ounces) of wine and the calorie sum is up to 420.

<u>Avocado & Rice Salad</u>

1 cup brown rice
3 tablespoons soy sauce
3 tablespoons rice wine
3 tablespoons vermouth
2 tablespoon sugar
1 cup cilantro leaves and tender stems
½ cup peanuts, toasted and roughly chopped
¼ cup pickled ginger, thinly sliced
4 scallions, thinly sliced
2 avocados, peeled, pitted, and thinly sliced
1 cucumber, halved lengthwise, sliced ¼ inch pieces
Zest and juice of 1 lime

1) Rinse rice in strainer under running cold water. Bring 12 cups water to a boil in a large pot with a tight-fitting lid over high heat. Add brown rice, stir once, and boil, uncovered, for 30 minutes. Pour rice into a strainer; cool to room temperature.

2) Sauce: Combine soy sauce, rice wine, vermouth, and sugar in a saucepan over medium-high heat; cook until sugar has dissolved, 3-5 minutes. Cool sauce slightly.

3) Combine rice, teriyaki sauce, cilantro, peanuts, ginger, scallions, avocados, cucumber, lime zest and juice in a bowl. Plate and garnish with cilantro.

<u>Serves 4</u>. About 410 Calories per serving

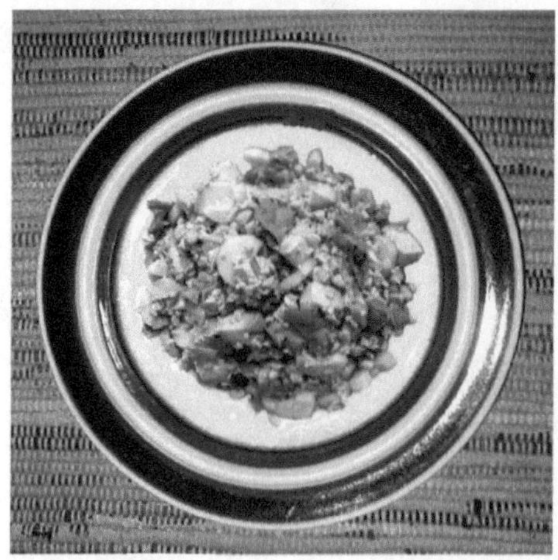

Note: The addition of a small whole-grain roll raises the total for this dish to 490 Calories.

Spinach & Fruit Side Salad

    4 ounces baby spinach
    3 ounces strawberries
    3 ounces blueberries
    3 ounces raspberries
    1½ tablespoons low-calorie salad dressing*

1) Rinse and drain spinach, strawberries, blueberries and raspberries.
2) Plate spinach. Add strawberries, blueberries and raspberries. Drizzle with 1½ tablespoons salad dressing.

Serves 4. About 100 Calories per serving.

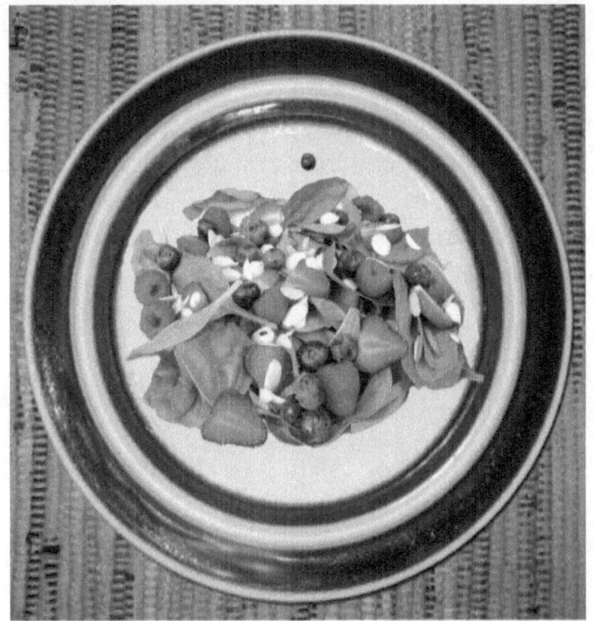

* Use low-calorie salad dressing that contains no more than 25 Calories per tablespoon.

Recipe 101

<u>Super Fruit Salad</u>

½ a medium seedless watermelon
1 medium cantaloupe
4 ounces raspberries
4 ounces blackberries
4 ounces blueberries
zest and juice of one lime
1 tablespoon honey
1 tablespoon water
1 tablespoon mint leaves, mince
4 to 8 mint leaves

1) Use a melon ball scoop or knife to create bite size pieces of watermelon and cantaloupe.
2) Add the melon to a large bowl. Add raspberries, blackberries, and blueberries to melon. Toss gently, so you don't crush berries.
3) Dressing: In a small bowl, combine zest and juice of one lime, honey, water, and minced mint leaves.
4) Drizzle dressing over fruit to coat. Use remaining mint leaves as garnish. Cover and chill before serving, about 2 hours.

<u>Serves 6</u>. About 180 Calories per serving.

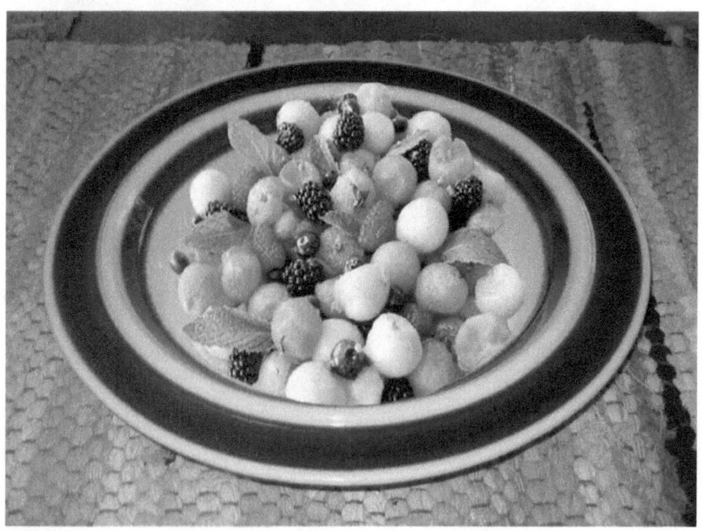

Tofu is an excellent non-animal high-protein food made from soybeans that is frequently linked with vegetarianism. Tofu comes in two basic varieties: soft or silken tofu and firm or regular tofu. Tofu has no taste but readily absorbs the flavor of other foods. Refrigerate tofu after you open a package and use it within four days.

Firm versions of tofu (well-drained) are used for kebabs, mock meats, and dishes requiring a consistency that holds together, while the softer tofu styles are used in desserts, soups, shakes, and sauces. Grated firm western tofu is sometimes used as a meat substitute and can be barbecued because it will hold together on a barbecue grill. Soft tofu is sometimes used as a dairy-free or low-calorie filler. Silken tofu may be used to replace cheese in certain dishes such as lasagna.

Most proteins are delicious even when seasoned simply with salt and pepper. Not tofu which most often tofu tastes bland. But you can turn it into a food you actually want to eat with the following tips.

Buying Tofu

Tofu is usually found in a refrigerated case in the produce department (fruit and vegetables) of most supermarkets. Some stores have tofu in the dairy section and others in stock it in health-food.

Preparing Tofu

1) Most tofu comes packed in water. But a water-logged block of tofu won't absorb a marinade or get crispy in a frying pan. The first thing to do is drain the block as much as possible. To drain it, slice the block and place the slices on a paper towel-lined baking sheet. Top tofu with more paper towels and then a heavy object. Let tofu sit at least one hour. Once drained, you can marinate the tofu or start cooking it.

2) After pressing, tofu is ready to absorb flavor. But the tofu still retains some water and oil and water don't mix. In most cases, use soy, citrus, or vinegar-based marinades instead.

3) Trying to get tofu crispy is difficult. Tossing tofu in cornstarch overcomes the difficulty. Place cornstarch in a bowl, add drained or marinated tofu pieces, and toss. A light coating is best.

4) To sear tofu, use sesame oil which can take the heat and doubles as a flavoring agent, giving the tofu a nutty flavor.

Leftover Tofu

Once a package of tofu is opened it will last about three days if refrigerated. You can freeze leftover tofu. Frozen tofu can last up to three months. And you can freeze any kind of tofu: silken, firm, or extra-firm. Just cut the tofu into cubes and freeze the cubes on a baking sheet. Once hard, store the tofu together in a freezer container. Thaw leftover tofu on a counter top during dinner prep. Thawed tofu can be cooked just as fresh tofu. But squeeze the tofu gently before cooking to eliminate extra moisture.

<u>Disclaimer</u>

This book offers general meal planning, nutrition and weight control information. It is not a medical manual and the author does not claim to be medically qualified. The material in this book is not intended to be a substitute for medical counseling. Everyone should have a medical checkup before beginning a weight loss program. Moreover, the physician conducting the medical exam should be made aware of and should approve the specific weight control program planned. Additionally, while the author and publisher have made every effort to ensure the accuracy of the information in this book, they make no representations or warranties regarding its accuracy or completeness. Further, neither the author nor publisher assume liability for any medical problems that might result from applying the methods in this book, or for any loss of profit, or any other commercial damages, including but not limited to special, incidental, consequential or other damages, and any such liability is hereby expressly disclaimed.

NoPaperPress eBooks and Paperbacks

100-Day Super Diet-1200 Cal*
100-Day Super Diet-1500 Cal*
100-Day No-Cooking Diet-1200 Cal*
100-Day No-Cooking Diet-1500 Cal*
90-Day Smart Diet-1200 Cal*
90-Day Smart Diet-1500 Cal*
90-Day No-Cooking Diet - 1200 Cal*
90-Day No-Cooking Diet - 1500 Cal*
90-Day Perfect Diet - 1200 Cal*
90-Day Perfect Diet - 1500 Cal*
60-Day Perfect Diet-1200 Cal*
60-Day Perfect Diet-1500 Cal*
50-Day Flex Diet-1200 Cal*
50-Day Flex Diet-1500 Cal*
30-Day Quick Diet - Women*
30-Day Quick Diet for Men*
30-Day No-Cooking Diet*
30-Day Diet - Women - Metric*
30-Day Diet for Men - Metric*
25 Day Easy Diet-1200 Cal*
25 Day Easy Diet-1500 Cal*
25-Day No-Cooking Diet
10-Day Express Diet
10-Day No-Cooking Diet*
7-Day Diet for Women*
7-Day Diet for Men*
7-Day No-Cooking Diets*
90-Day Gluten-Free Diet-1200 Cal*
90-Day Gluten-Free Diet-1500 Cal*
30-Day Gluten-Free Quick Diet*
30-Day Gluten-Free No-Cooking Diet*
7-Day Diet for Women - Metric*
7-Day Diet for Men - Metric
7-Day Gluten-Free Express Diet*
7-Day Gluten-Free No-Cooking Diet*
90-Day Vegetarian Diet-1200 Cal*
90-Day Vegetarian Diet-1500 Cal*
30-Day Vegetarian Diet*
7-Day Vegetarian Diet*
Weight Loss for Women*
Weight Loss for Women - Metric
Weight Loss for Women - UK
Weight Loss for Men*
Maximum Weight Loss - 1200 Cal*
Maximum Weight Loss - 1500 Cal*

Weight Loss for Men - Metric*
Maximum Weight Loss- 1200 Cal*
Maximum Weight Loss- 1500 Cal*
Weight Control - U.S. Edition*
Weight Control - Metric. Edition
Prof Weight Control Women - U.S.
Prof Weight Control Women - Metric
Prof Weight Control Men - U.S.
Prof Weight Control Men - Metric
Weight Maintenance - U.S. Ed*
Weight Maintenance - Metric. Ed*
Weight Maintenance - UK Ed
Weight Loss for Senior Men*
Weight Loss for Senior Women*
Eat Smart - U.S. Edition*
Eat Smart - Metric Edition
30-Day Mediterranean Diet
Exercise Smart - U.S. Edition*
Exercise Smart - Metric Edition
Exercise Smart - UK Edition*
Total Fitness - U.S. Edition
Total Fitness - Metric Edition
Total Fitness - UK Edition
Total Fitness for Women-U.S. Ed*
Total Fitness for Women - Metric
Total Fitness for Women - UK Ed
Total Fitness for Men - U.S. Ed*
Total Fitness for Men- Metric Ed*
Total Fitness for Men - UK Ed
Senior Fitness - U.S. Edition*
Senior Fitness - Metric Edition*
Senior Fitness - UK Edition*
Computer Diet - U.S. Edition*
Computer Diet - Metric Ed*
Reliable Weight Loss - U.S. Ed
101 Weight Loss Tips*
101 Healthy Eating Tips*
101 Lifelong Fitness Tips*
101 Weight Maintenance Tips
101 Weight Loss Recipes
101 GF Weight Loss Recipes
101 Veggie Weight Loss Recipes*
30-Day Mediterranean Diet*
90-Day Mediterranean Diet - 1200 Cal*
90-Day Mediterranean Diet - 1500 Cal*

* These titles are available as both ebooks and paperbacks. Our ebooks are sold by Amazon, Apple, Google, Barnes & Noble and Kobo, but our paperbacks are only sold by Amazon.